# The Principles and Practice of Electrical Epilation

*Second Edition*

Sheila Godfrey, DRE, FBAE, BABTAC

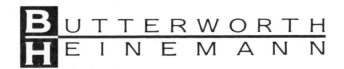

Butterworth-Heinemann
Linacre House, Jordan Hill, Oxford OX2 8DP
225 Wildwood Avenue, Woburn, MA 01801-2041
A division of Reed Educational and Professional Publishing Ltd

A member of the Reed Elsevier plc group

OXFORD    AUCKLAND    BOSTON
JOHANNESBURG    MELBOURNE    NEW DELHI

First published 1992
Reprinted 1993 (twice), 1994, 1995 (twice)
Second edition 1996
Reprinted 1997, 1998, 1999

**British Library Cataloguing in Publication Data**
Godfrey, Sheila
Principles and Practice of Electrical Epilation - 2nd ed.
1. Hair - removal   2. Electrolysis in surgery
I. Title
617.4'779

ISBN 0 7506 2924 X

Typeset by Scribe Design, Gillingham, Kent
Printed and bound in Great Britain by The Bath Press, Bath

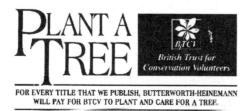

FOR EVERY TITLE THAT WE PUBLISH, BUTTERWORTH-HEINEMANN
WILL PAY FOR BTCV TO PLANT AND CARE FOR A TREE.

# Contents

# Introduction

The purpose of this book is to provide up-to-date information on all aspects of electro-epilation for both practising electrolysists and students studying for any of the following epilation qualifications:

- National/Scottish Vocational Qualification Level 3 (N/SVQ).
- British Technical Education Centre (BTEC).
- Confederation of International Beauty Therapy and Cosmetology (CIBTAC).
- City and Guilds of London Institute (CGLI).
- British Association of Electrolysists Ltd (BAE).

Many changes have taken place in this field during the last twenty years, yet up-to-date information has so far not been available in any single text. The wide-ranging changes that have taken place include:

- Improved standards of training.
- Health and Safety at Work Act 1974.
- The advent of pre-sterilized disposable needles.
- Local Government Miscellaneous Provisions Act 1982.
- Changes relating to technology in the development and manufacturing of equipment.
- The arrival of AIDS.
- The rising incidence of hepatitis B.
- The identification of hepatitis C, D and E.
- The introduction of Blend epilation into the UK.
- The lifting of trade barriers between member countries of the European Community in 1992.
- The introduction of the National/Scottish Vocational Qualification Level 3 in Electrical Epilation in Britain.

Knowledge of allied subjects such as endocrinology, hygiene, anatomy, physiology and electricity is essential to a thorough understanding of why hair growth occurs and how this problem, which causes distress to very many people, can be treated safely and efficiently.

**Companies consulted**

Allenbrooke Kingsley Mills, Chartered Accountants, Birmingham
Ballet Needles, Paris
Carlton Professional, Taylor Reeson Laboratories, Sussex
Continental Trades and Industry, Amsterdam, Holland
E. A. Ellison, Coventry
Hairdressing and Beauty Equipment Centre, London
Hairdressers Insurance Bureau, Haywards Heath, Sussex
International Hair Route Magazine, Ontario
Lloyds Bank Plc, England
Specialist Computer Centres, Birmingham
Solihull Hospital, Microbiology Department

# Acknowledgements

I wish to express my thanks to the many people who so willingly provided information for both editions of this book.

My particular thanks go to the late Rod Fabes and his engineers, Paul Atherton and Chris Johnson of Carlton Professional, Joseph Asch of Ballet Needles, Paris for his valuable input into this second edition, particularly in relation to the provision of photographs, and Romano Scavo of CTI Holland, for his help with technical information and photographs. James Paisner of Synoptics Products for information on sterilization requirements/standards in the USA, and Derek Copperthwaite of *International Hair Route Magazine* for providing material on the history of the epilation needle.

Special gratitude is due to Kenneth Morris for his meticulous attention to detail and for the many hours spent checking the manuscript: also Bill Peberdy, David Bragg, Pauline Perks, Kay Judd, Penny Turvey and Dawn Mernagh for their support and encouragement. Thanks are due also to Rita Roberts for her sympathetic teaching and support throughout the years and my American colleague John Fantz of California for sharing his knowledge on the history and development of Blend epilation.

Photographs supplied by:

Carlton Professional, Figure 13.5.
Ballet Needles, cover photograph and Figures 9.7 and 14.4.
Hairdressing and Beauty Equipment Centre, Figures 13.5 and 18.7.
John Fantz, Figures 11.1, 13.1 and 13.2.
Joseph Asch, Figures 13.15, 13.16, 13.17 and 14.1.

# 1 Skin

The skin is the largest organ of the body, and skin has many functions. It serves as a protective, waterproof covering for the body, it aids in regulation of body temperature, and it is the principal area for the sense of touch.

The practising electrolysist should be fully conversant with the anatomy and physiology of skin, and should be able to recognize the differences between a healthy skin and one suffering from disease or disorders.

The skin consists of three main layers: (a) epidermis, (b) dermis and (c) subcutaneous layer (see Figure 1.1). The epidermis can then be further divided into several more layers, as illustrated in Figure 1.2.

There are a number of appendages of the skin which need to be considered. These are shown in Figure 1.3.

## The epidermis

This is the topmost layer of the skin. It is non-vascular and consists of stratified epithelium. The thickness varies from one area to another; it is thinner on the lips and eyelids and thicker on the palms of the hand and soles of the feet.

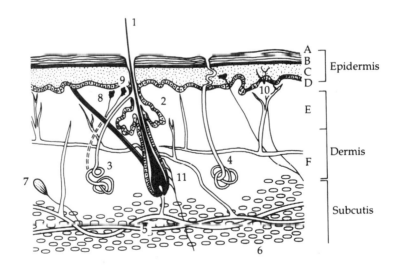

A Stratum corneum ⎤
B Stratum granulosum ⎥ Epidermis
C Prickle cell layer ⎥
D Basal cell layer ⎦
E Papillary layer ⎤ Dermis
F Reticular layer ⎦

1 Hair in hair follicle
2 Sebaceous gland
3 Apocrine sweat gland
4 Eccrine sweat gland
5 Blood vessels
6 Fat cells
7 Pacinian corpuscle–pressure/touch
8 Kraus bulbs–cold
9 Raffini–heat
10 Free nerve endings–pain
11 Nerve endings to follicle

**Figure 1.1** Cross-section of the skin

1

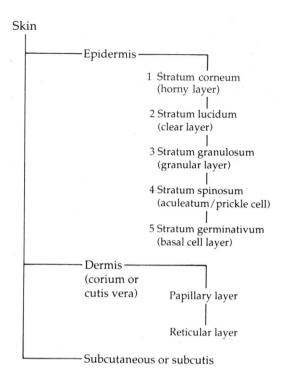

**Figure 1.2** Layers of the skin

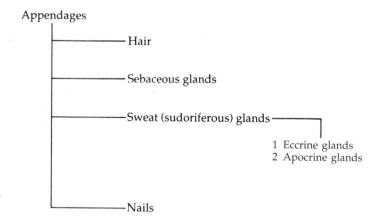

**Figure 1.3** Appendages of the skin

**The stratum germinativum**

Also known as the basal cell layer, this is the deepest layer of the epidermis. This layer and the stratum spinosum together are known as the *Malpighian layer*, or *Stratum malpighii*. The germinativum is closely moulded on to the papillary layer of the dermis below. The cells are keratinocytes, contain nuclei and are therefore capable of cell division. They are larger than cells in the upper layers, and are columnar in shape. The contents are soft, opaque and granular. Cells contain melanocytes.

**The stratum spinosum**

This is also known as the prickle cell layer (or the stratum aculeatum). It is situated directly adjacent to the stratum granulosum. Here the cells are covered with numerous fibrils which connect the surfaces of the cells. These cells are known as prickle cells. Between the cells are fine intercellular clefts which allow the passage of lymph corpuscles. Pigment granules may be found here. Cells have flattened slightly.

**The stratum granulosum**

This lies immediately under the stratum lucidum, and consists of granular cells. The granules contain a substance known as keratohyaline, which is an intermediate substance in the formation of keratin. Nuclei and other cell contents begin to disappear. (The granules consist of a substance called eleidin which is the intermediate substance in the formation of horn. (*Grays Anatomy,* page 1138.)

**The stratum lucidum**

This layer, which is present only in the palms of the hands and soles of the feet, consists of flattened, closely packed cells. Traces of flattened nuclei may be found. The cells are transparent, which allows the passage of sunlight to the deeper layers.

**The stratum corneum**

Also known as the horny layer, this is the topmost layer, consisting of flattened, keratinized cells, which are horny, hard, and do not contain a nucleus. These outer cells are constantly being shed and replaced from the lower layers.

# The dermis

The dermis, also known as the *corium* or *cutis vera,* is situated immediately below the epidermis. It contains blood vessels, lymph vessels and nerves. This is the largest layer of the skin and consists of two parts: the upper papillary layer, and the lower reticular layer.

**The papillary layer**

This is situated on the free surface of the reticular layer and consists of a number of small, highly sensitive projections known as papillae. The papillae are composed of very small, closely interlacing bundles of fibrillated tissue. Within this tissue is a capillary loop. Tactile corpuscles can be found in some of these papillae.

**The reticular layer**

This forms the bulk of the dermis and lies immediately below the papillary layer. The majority of the collagen and elastin fibres are found here. Fibroblasts are spindle-shaped cells which are responsible for the production of collagen and elastin fibres. 'Mast cells' are responsible for the release of histamine and heparin. The function of histamine is to dilate blood vessels, and the function of heparin is to prevent blood from clotting. The typical mast cell is large, rounded or spindle shaped with one, or occasionally two, nuclei.

The dermis is composed of connective tissue which contains a ground substance or matrix that contains most of the skin's water content, in which, are suspended:

1  Cells (fibroblasts and mast cells).
2  Fibres – collagen, elastin and reticulin.

There are three different connective tissues found in the dermis. These are:

1  White fibrous tissue/collagen.
2  Yellow elastic tissue/elastin.
3  Reticulin.

*Collagen fibres, also known as white fibrous tissue,* form 75 per cent of the total connective tissue. The fibres are embedded in a ground substance of colloidal gel. Fibroblasts are interspersed between the bundles of collagen. Collagen gives the skin its toughness and resilience.

*Elastin, or yellow fibres,* forms 4 per cent of the connective tissue. These fibres run parallel or obliquely to the collagen and enclose the bundles. Elastin gives the skin its elasticity.

*Reticulin fibres* are thought to ensure stability between the dermis and epidermis.

Structures found within the dermis are:

1  Sebaceous glands.
2  Sweat (sudoriferous) glands.
3  Arrector pili muscles.
4  Hair follicles.

## Sebaceous glands

Sebaceous glands are situated within the dermis, with their ducts opening into the hair follicle. Occasionally, some may open directly on to the skin's surface. They are absent in the palms of the hands and soles of the feet. Each gland is constructed of a single duct which ends in a cluster of secretory saccules similar to a bunch of grapes in appearance.

Sebaceous glands are highly sensitive to androgens, which stimulate the growth of the gland and the production of sebum. Sebum production is increased at puberty and decreases with age. It is secreted via the hair follicle on to the skin's surface. The purpose of sebum is to keep the hair pliable and to lubricate the skin. It is responsible for making the skin waterproof and plays a major role in the maintenance of the 'acid mantle' (see page 6). Sebum contains fatty acids, esters and other substances.

## Sweat (sudoriferous) glands

Sweat glands, more correctly termed 'sudoriferous glands' are found all over the body surface. Their function is to regulate body heat through the evaporation of sweat on the skin's surface and also to excrete a small amount of waste products. Sweat glands can be divided into eccrine and apocrine glands.

Eccrine glands are present in large numbers – between two and five million in total. They are found in all parts of the skin with the exception of mucous membranes.

The eccrine gland (see Figure 1.4) is a down-growth of the epidermis which reaches into the deeper layers of the dermis where it forms a coiled ball known as the glomerulus. The duct is straight in the upper dermis, and becomes twisted, like a corkscrew, in the epidermis.

The secretion from eccrine glands is a clear, watery fluid consisting of 99–99.5 per cent water, together with some chlorides, lactic acid and urea.

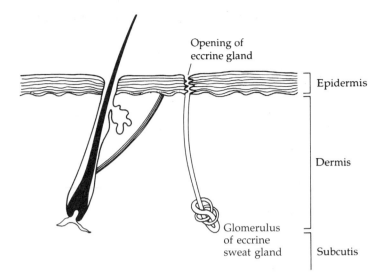

**Figure 1.4** Eccrine
sweat gland

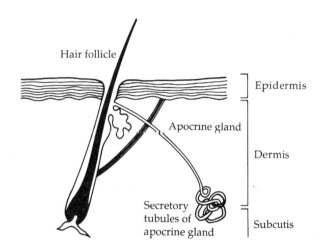

**Figure 1.5** Apocrine
gland

The apocrine glands (Figure 1.5) are larger than eccrine glands, and are usually attached to hair follicles. Their ducts open into the hair follicle – only occasionally do they open directly on to the skin's surface. They are coiled, tubular glands with a duct leading down to a coil of secretory tubules. Apocrine glands are found in the axilla, groin, and around the nipples. They are under hormonal control and become active at puberty. Stimulation is brought about by stress, fright, pain or sexual activity.

Secretion from these glands is a sterile, whitish fluid which contains proteins, carbohydrates and other substances.

# Functions of the skin

The skin performs a number of functions. These are illustrated in Figure 1.6.

## *Secretion*

The secretion of sebum on to the skin's surface helps to lubricate the hair and skin, keeping them soft and pliable. Sebum is responsible for the

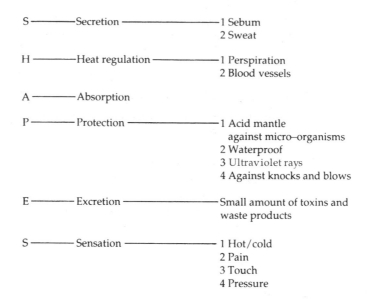

**Figure 1.6** Functions of the skin

formation of the acid mantle, and provides a waterproof film on the epidermis. Sudoriferous glands secrete sweat on to the surface via the ducts.

### Heat regulation

This is maintained in two ways. Blood carries heat. When there is too much heat in the body the cutaneous blood vessels dilate releasing heat, some of which is lost by radiation. This heat is responsible for the evaporation of sweat on the skin's surface, which has a cooling effect.

When heat needs to be conserved the reverse action takes place, with blood vessels constricting, so keeping the heat within the body. There is a reduction in the amount of sweat secreted by the sweat (sudoriferous) glands.

### Absorption

The use of patches impregnated with drugs or hormones shows without doubt that the skin is capable of absorbing some substances. Indeed hormone replacement therapy is often administered in this way, with patches containing oestrogen attached to the skin and changed at regular intervals according to the doctor's instructions.

### Protection

The skin protects the body in several ways. Melanocytes, found in the epidermis, produce melanin which helps to protect the skin from the harmful effects of ultraviolet rays.

The 'acid mantle' refers to a fine film of sebum and sweat found on the surface of the skin. The function of the acid mantle is to inhibit the growth of bacteria. The pH scale is measured on a scale from 0 to 14, with 7 being neutral. The lower the number the higher the acidity. The normal pH of white skin is between 4.5 and 6. The acid mantle is often destroyed by the over-enthusiastic use of soaps and harsh detergents.

The subcutaneous layer gives protection from knocks and blows by acting as a buffer.

The horny nature of keratinized cells in the epidermis prevents the entry of harsh chemicals.

**Figure 1.7** The pH scale

| 0 | 1 | 2 | 3 | 4 | 5 | 6 | 7 | 8 | 9 | 10 | 11 | 12 | 13 | 14 |
|---|---|---|---|---|---|---|---|---|---|----|----|----|----|----|

Acid       N |       Alkaline

*Excretion*

Small amounts of waste products are eliminated from the body on to the skin's surface via sweat. The amount of waste matter increases during times of stress or ill health.

*Sensation*

The skin is the principal seat of sensation. Due to the abundant supply of sensory nerves contained within the papillary layer of the dermis, it is possible for the skin to respond to heat, cold, pain, and pressure. The nerve supply also surrounds the hair follicle, arrector pili muscle and sweat glands.

Nerves within the skin end either in a corpuscle or free endings. It is the free-ending nerves which are responsible for the sense of pain. Those ending in corpuscles are of three types:

1 Pacinnian – responsible for touch or pressure.
2 Krause bulbs – responsible for sensation of cold.
3 Organs of Raffini – responsible for feeling heat.

Meissner corpuscles are unique sensory receptors found only in the hands, feet and digits.

*Formation of vitamin D*

Vitamin D is formed by the action of ultraviolet light on dehydrocholesterol in the skin. Vitamin D aids in the formation and maintenance of healthy bone.

*Natural moisturizing factor*

The function of the natural moisturizing factor is to aid in the prevention of loss of moisture from the epidermis. As the cells within the skin structures move up towards the surface, moisture is pressed out of the cell which results in each cell being coated with a sticky intercellular glue, thereby holding the stratum corneum together.

# Black skins

There are a number of differences between the structure of black and white skins which should be considered when giving electrical epilation treatment.

*Sweat (sudoriferous) glands*

In black races the sudoriferous glands are larger and more numerous. The glomerulus is rounder but not as coiled. The secretory duct which opens on to the surface of the skin is longer and more noticeable.

There are a larger number of eccrine glands per square cm, with the pH balance being between 3.5 and 5.6.

In black races melanin pigment is found in the glomerulus and sometimes in the wall of the excretory duct.

*Sebaceous glands*

The sebaceous glands are not only larger and more numerous, but approximately 10 per cent open directly on to the skin's surface with the other 90 per cent opening into the hair follicle.

**Pigmentation**

The colour of the skin is affected by several substances:

1 Melanin.
2 Melanoid.
3 Carotene.
4 Haemoglobin.
5 Oxyhaemoglobin.

It is important to remember when treating black skins with electrical epilation that it is not easy to detect erythema. Therefore care must be taken to ensure that the skin does not become over treated due to too much heat being applied in any one area.

**The stratum corneum**

In a black skin this is thicker than in a white skin, with black skin desquamating more easily. Pigmentary granules are present in the desquamating cells of black skin but not of white skin (H. Pierantoni, *Essential Notions of Black Skin*, 1977).

**Keloids**

These are more frequently found on black skins. A keloid is an excessive formation of scar tissue at the site of an injury to the skin. It is essential that the electrolysist should discuss this possibility during the consultation prior to giving any treatment. Keloids can continue to grow and harden for several months after the initial injury.

**Asian skin**

Asian skin is normally finer in texture than black skin. Hair growth tends to be dense but fine and dark. Follicles are inclined to be small and straight. This skin is prone to sensitivity during treatment, care must be taken to avoid over treating any one area. Excess application of heat, or scarring, tends to leave dark pigmentation patches which are slow to fade.

**Oriental skin**

Oriental skin is prone to pigmentation, pit marks and discolouration due to exposure to heat and ultraviolet irradiation.

# Review questions

1 Name and describe the layers of the epidermis.
2 Name and describe the layers of the dermis.
3 Draw a clear fully labelled diagram of the skin.
4 List the appendages of the skin.
5 Name and describe the connective tissues of the dermis.
6 Give the location and function of the sebaceous glands.
7 Describe the difference between eccrine glands and apocrine glands.
8 Explain the functions of the skin.
9 What is meant by the term acid mantle of the skin?
10 What is the normal pH of the skin?
11 State the importance of the correct pH balance.
12 Describe the main differences between the structure of black and Caucasian (white) skin.
13 List the substances that affect the colour of the skin.

# 2 Dermatology

Electrolysists will find during the course of their professional life that knowledge of the skin's structure and function is not enough. The skin is the largest organ of the body and in many instances reflects the health of the individual. The electrolysist should therefore:

1  be able to recognize the different skin lesions;
2  be able to identify the most common skin diseases;
3  know the causes of these diseases;
4  be able to recognize when a disease is contra-indicated to electro-epilation;
5  know when to refer the client for further investigation by the medical profession.

Many skin conditions present similar lesions. Thorough examination in a good light is essential, as is careful questioning, which should include family background. In a number of instances accurate diagnosis is not possible without referral to the medical profession for further investigation. Guttate psoriasis and pityriasis rosea show many similarities and can easily be confused. In the early stages of pityriasis rosea the herald patch may be mistaken for ringworm at the initial inspection.

The health and condition of the skin is affected by a number of internal and external influences:

- *Hormonal* – low oestrogen levels cause the skin to become dry and lose collagen content. Androgens cause the skin to become oily. Steroid creams used over a prolonged period of time may result in thinning of the skin structures.
- *Allergies* – may be caused by food intolerances, alcohol, drugs such as aspirin and penicillin, cosmetic preparations, perfume, lanolin, preservatives and certain chemicals such as hair dyes.
- *Environment* – poor hygiene, exposure to ultraviolet light, humidity which affects pH balance, and central heating which may cause excessive dryness.
- *Genetic predisposition* – for example eczema
- *Nutritional deficiencies* – resulting in lack of essential vitamins and minerals, e.g. low levels of vitamin A leave the skin dry, insufficient vitamin C affects the strength of capillary walls which means that the skin bruises easily.

Stress over a prolonged period of time also has a detrimental effect on the skin, fine lines or dehydration may develop. Excess sebum may be produced due to increased levels of androgens, which in turn may also trigger increased hair growth.

## Common skin lesions

Skin lesions show alterations in the appearance of the skin. Depending on the severity, lesions are classified as primary, secondary or tertiary. The terms used to describe changes in the skin are shown in table 2.1.

**Table 2.1**

| | |
|---|---|
| Macule | Flat, small patch of increased pigmentation or discolouration, e.g. a freckle. |
| Papule | Small, raised elevation on the skin, less than 1 cm in diameter, which may be red in colour, e.g. acne and rosacea. |
| Pustule | Small, raised elevation of the skin which contains pus, seen in acne and rosacea. |
| Nodule | A well-defined, solid lump more than 1 cm in diameter, seen in boils and rodent ulcers. |
| Plaque | A well-defined, disc-shaped elevated area of skin, seen in psoriasis. |
| Vesicle | Small lesion containing fluid, i.e. small blisters seen in herpes simplex, herpes zoster and impetigo. |
| Bulla | Large lesion, more than 2–3 cm in diameter, containing fluid, i.e. blister. |
| Comedone | May be closed or open. This lesion is a collection of sebum, keratinized cells and certain waste substances which accumulate in the entrance of a hair follicle. An open comedone is a blackhead contained within the follicle, whereas a closed comedone, or whitehead, is trapped underneath the skin's surface. Closed comedones do have a small opening on the surface of the skin. |
| Milia | Small accumulation of fatty substances under the skin, often seen around the eyes and on the cheeks of dry skin. |
| Ulcer | A loss of epidermis (frequently with loss of underlying dermis and subcutis). Seen in a rodent ulcer. |
| Scale | Visible flakes of skin on the surface of the epidermis, seen in psoriasis. |
| Crust | Also referred to as a scab, this is an accumulation of dried fluid, serum or pus on the surface of the skin, seen in impetigo. |
| Fissure | Crack in the skin's surface, e.g. chapped lips which can be painful. |
| Excoriation | A secondary superficial ulceration which is due to scratching. |
| Wheal | Well-defined raised area of cutaneous oedema, white in the centre with a red edge, seen in urticaria. |
| Scar | Appears during the healing process. Skin tissue may be smooth and shiny or form a depression in the surface, e.g. an ice-pick scar seen in acne. |
| Telangiectasia | Persistent vasodilation of the capillaries in the skin. |
| Keloid | Over-growth of scar tissue with a raised, shiny appearance. |

## Changes in skin colour and appearance

*Hyperkeratosis:* refers to excess keratinization of cells, or over-growth of horny cells, e.g. scales and plaques found in psoriasis.

*Erythema:* general redness of the skin due to temporary or permanent vasodilation.

*Hyper-pigmentation:* describes an excess or increase in skin pigmentation, e.g. chloasma, lentigo.

*Hypo-pigmentation:* describes loss of pigmentation, e.g. vitiligo.

## Causes

Skin diseases and disorders may occur as a result of one of the following:

1 Bacterial infection.
2 Viral infection.
3 Fungal infection.
4 Parasites.
5 Exposure to allergens.
6 Hereditary/genetic predisposition.
7 Pigmentation abnormalities.
8 Hormonal influences.
9 Stress related.
10 Carcinogenic/cancer.

### Bacterial infections
#### Boils

Boils are caused by a staphylococcal infection of the hair follicle. The area becomes red, swollen and painful. Heat and oedema are present. After a short period of time the centre fills with pus and eventually bursts. A scar frequently develops after the boil has healed.

Common sites for the development of boils are the axilla, the back of the neck, the buttocks and thighs. Their appearance is a sign of lower resistance to infection due to being tired and run down.

Carbuncles develop when a number of boils appear in close proximity to one another.

#### Erythrasma

Erythrasma is a bacterial infection produced by a gram-positive bacillus, *Corynebacterium inutissimum*. Common sites for the development of erythrasma are the axilla, groin and submammary regions, but the commonest site colonized by this bacteria is in between the toes.

The characteristics of erythrasma are the appearance of marginated brown areas with a fine, branny surface scale. Symptoms can be aggravated by increased temperature, perspiration and scratching of the area due to irritation.

#### Impetigo

Impetigo is a superficial, contagious, inflammatory disease caused by streptococcal and staphylococcal bacteria. It is commonly seen on the face and around the ears. Weeping vesicles dry to form honey-coloured crusts. The bacteria can be transmitted by dirty fingernails and towels. Impetigo may also arise as a secondary infection from an existing condition such as scabies.

### Viral infections

Conditions caused by a viral infection include warts, herpes simplex and herpes zoster, all of which are contagious.

#### Warts

Warts appear in several forms. They are well-defined, benign tumours which vary in size and shape. The *common wart* varies in size from a pinhead to the size of a pea. The surface can be smooth or rough. These warts are usually found on the fingers and hands. *Plane warts* are found on the face, forehead, back of hands or front of knees. They are smooth in texture with a flat top. The *plantar wart* is the size of a pea, or a little larger. These are found on the sole of the foot and may be very painful. This type of wart is also called a verruca. The *filiform wart* hangs down from the skin's surface and may grow up to 6 mm in length. These are quite thick in diameter. The neck is the most usual site for this type of wart.

**Herpes simplex**

Herpes simplex (also referred to as cold sores) is normally found on the face and around the lips. The onset is quite rapid, beginning with an itching sensation, shortly followed by erythema and groups of vesicles. Crusts form where the vesicles weep. The condition clears up in approximately two to three weeks, but will reappear in the same area in times of stress, ill health or exposure to sunlight.

**Herpes zoster**

Herpes zoster is also known as shingles. It is caused by a virus closely related to the chicken-pox virus. The condition is very painful due to acute inflammation of one or more peripheral nerves. The pain may persist for up to 18 months. The lesions resemble herpes simplex, with erythema and vesicles along the line of a nerve. Areas affected include the chest and back and along the trigeminal nerve of the face.

**Fungal infections**

Fungal infections include tinea pedis, tinea capitis, tinea corporis and pityriasis versicolor, also known as tinea pityriasis.

Tinea or ringworm is caused by a superficial fungus which lives on the skin and feeds off dead horny cells. The fungi digest keratin. There are several forms of fungal infection, but the three which are of most interest to the electrolysist are tinea corporis, affecting the body, tinea capitis, affecting the scalp, and tinea pedis – athlete's foot – affecting the feet.

**Tinea corporis**

Also known as ringworm of the body, this exhibits lesions which begin as small red papules that gradually increase in size to form a ring. These lesions, which vary in shape from round to oval, gradually clear in the centre as they increase in size. However some lesions do not clear from the centre but appear as red, scaly plaques.

**Tinea capitis**

This particular fungal infection affects both the hair and the scalp. Lesions appear as small oval patches on the scalp. The hairs break off near to the skin's surface, which has a scaly base.

**Tinea pedis**

Tinea pedis, more commonly referred to as athlete's foot, is highly contagious and can easily be acquired from damp places such as swimming pools, showers or saunas. A sign of athlete's foot is the appearance of flaking skin between the toes which becomes soft and soggy. The skin may also split and the condition is sometimes uncomfortable. Occasionally the soles of the feet are affected.

**Pityriasis versicolor (tinea versicolor)**

Pityriasis versicolor is a *superficial* fungal infection which affects the back, chest and axilla. This condition develops gradually and can be recognized by the appearance of well-defined fawn or coffee-coloured lesions with fine branny scales, on the neck, shoulders, upper trunk and upper arms.

## Infestations by insects
### Scabies

Scabies, caused by the sarcoptes scabiei parasite, is a contagious parasitic infection caused by the itch mite. The female mite (arcarus) burrows into the horny layer of the skin where she lays her eggs. The eggs hatch after three to four days, and the larvae gravitate from their burrows into the adjacent hair follicles. After approximately 17 days the adult mites emerge and the whole cycle starts again. The adult female mite may live in her burrow for between six to eight weeks.

A characteristic lesion in scabies is the burrow, a white or greyish zigzag line, which may be slightly curved and scaly, which varies in length between 0.5 cm and 1 cm. Vesicles may be visible at one end of the lesion. The onset of this condition is gradual, the first noticeable signs being severe itching which is usually worse at night. A generalized rash may then appear, with irritation becoming noticeable during the day. Papules, pustules, excoriations and crusted lesions may also develop. Common sites for this infestation are the ulnar borders of the wrists, palms of the hands and between the fingers. Other sites which may be affected are the axillary folds, the buttocks, breasts in the female and external genitalia in the male.

### Pediculosis (lice)

Pediculosis is also a contagious parasitic infestation, where the lice live off blood sucked from the skin. The female louse lays numerous eggs during her one-month life-span.

Nits are small, white oval eggs which are attached to the hair. They may be moved up or down a hair but cannot be removed sideways. After six to ten days these nits hatch into larvae, developing into fully-grown lice within one to two weeks.

Head lice (pediculosis capitis) are frequently seen in very young children who become infested at school. The condition spreads very quickly and can only be controlled by thorough treatment. The lice make no distinction between class or race and are happiest in clean hair. If not dealt with swiftly this condition may lead to secondary infection as a result of scratching, e.g. impetigo.

Body lice (pediculosis corporis) are rarely seen today. They usually occur on a person with poor personal hygiene. They live and reproduce in the seams and fibres of clothing, leaving only to feed from the skin. Lesions may appear as papules, scabs, and in severe cases pigmented, dry scaly skin. Secondary bacterial infection is often present.

### Eczema/dermatitis

The terms eczema and dermatitis are synonymous, in other words both terms may be used to describe the same condition. Eczema is derived from the Greek term 'ekzein' meaning to break out or boil over; 'dermatitis' means inflammation of the derma or skin. Both terms relate to a condition which varies from a mild to a chronic inflammatory state.

Eczema may be due to genetic predisposition, or to internal or external influences. When genetic predisposition is the root cause it is not unusual to find a history of asthma and/or hay fever in the family.

Clinical signs of eczema begin with small, itchy patches of erythema which may gradually increase in size. Oedema, fissures (cracks), scales and hyperkeratosis are other symptoms associated with this condition. In severe cases the skin weeps where fissures are present or where the surface has been scratched.

| | |
|---|---|
| *Contact dermatitis/eczema* | This is caused by a primary irritant which causes a reaction in susceptible individuals. The reaction may occur after a short exposure to an irritant or may build up over a period of time after repeated contact.

Substances which cause this type of eczema include: acids; alkalis; solvents; cosmetic preparations, in particular perfume and lanolin; detergents; nickel, e.g. ear-rings and suspenders; household polishes, plus certain house and garden plants, e.g. primulas, tulips, chrysanthemums and celery. Lesions are normally localized to the area of contact. |
| *Allergic dermatitis/eczema* | This is generally more widespread and does not appear immediately after the first exposure to the irritant or allergen. The individual gradually builds up a sensitivity to substances such as perfume or certain dairy products. Cow's milk is a common cause of eczema in children. Once sensitivity to an allergen has developed, further contact, even after a period of weeks or months, will result in the recurrence of eczema.

The sites most commonly affected are the hands and feet, but any area of the body may react when exposed to the offending substance. As with contact dermatitis, erythema is present and the skin becomes itchy with a build up of scales. In chronic cases small blisters, hyperkeratosis and fissures develop. Scratching will aggravate the condition. |
| *Seborrhoeic dermatitis (seborrhoeic eczema)* | Seborrhoeic dermatitis is a mild to chronic inflammatory disease of hairy areas well supplied with sebaceous glands. An increase in sebum production with an alteration in chemical composition may or may not be present. Common sites for this condition are the scalp, the face, axilla, sub-mammary folds and the groin.

The skin may appear to have a grey tinge or be dirty-yellow in colour. The onset of the condition is gradual. Clinical signs may show slight redness and scaling of the naso-labial folds, dandruff in the eyebrows and possibly deep-seated pustules affecting the follicles in the beard area of the adult male. When the scalp is affected greasy scales or dry, scaly plaques will be seen. |
| **Psoriasis** | Psoriasis is a chronic inflammatory condition of the skin. Although the cause is not known there is no doubt that a genetic factor exists. Any age group can be affected, but it very rarely appears in children under five years of age. Psoriasis is aggravated by stress, bacterial throat infection and trauma to the skin, but is improved by exposure to sunlight.

This disorder can be recognized by the development of well-defined red plaques which vary in size and shape, covered by white or silvery scales. When the scales are removed the surface underneath will be smooth and red and will show pin-point bleeding. The edges of plaques are well defined.

Any area of the body may develop psoriasis, but the most commonly affected sites are the extensor surfaces, chest, abdomen, face, elbows, knees and nails. |
| **Pityriasis rosea** | Pityriasis rosea begins with the appearance of the herald patch seven to ten days prior to development of other lesions. The herald patch usually appears on the trunk. This initial lesion presents itself as a scaly patch with a slightly raised edge which clears in the centre. At this stage it is possible to confuse pityriasis rosea with tinea corporis. The disease has no known cause. It can be termed self-limiting, and usually runs its course within six weeks. |

Clinical signs are oval-shaped lesions with well-defined edges and a scaly surface. Macules and papules may also be present. Pityriasis rosea appears mainly on the trunk and very rarely affects the face, hands or feet.

**Acne vulgaris**

Acne vulgaris is a condition which causes much emotional stress and embarrassment. Onset is gradual, appearing most frequently at puberty and persisting for some considerable time. Acne vulgaris rarely lasts beyond the age of 30. Salon treatments, while not making any claims to cure the problem, do help to keep lesions under control and scarring to a minimum. Exposure to ultraviolet light in the form of sunbeds and sunlight helps to improve the condition. The condition is often aggravated during the week before menstruation, during times of stress, e.g. examinations, and in humid climates. Areas most affected are the face, chest and back.

Acne vulgaris is due to a defect in the sebaceous glands which leads to over-production of sebum. It is primarily androgen induced and may indicate hyper-sensitivity of the sebaceous glands to circulating hormones.

Clinical features are the presence of comedones – both open and closed – papules, pustules, cysts, scars and hyperkeratosis of the horny layer. The skin is usually oily due to excess sebum on the epidermis. Ice-pick or keloid scars may also develop in susceptible individuals.

**Sebaceous cysts**

Sebaceous cysts are round, nodular lesions with a smooth, shiny surface which develop from a sebaceous gland. They are usually found on the face, neck, scalp and back. The cause is unknown. They are situated in the dermis and vary in size from 5 to 50 mm. The lesion is surrounded by fibrous connective tissue. Cysts contain masses of disintegrating epithelial cells, the contents of which are soft and cheesy.

**Rosacea**

The cause of rosacea is not known but it usually affects adults of both sexes from the age of 30 years onwards, although it is more frequently seen from the age of 45 years. Aggravating factors are heat, hot spicy foods, hot drinks, alcohol, emotional stress, menopause, cold winds and sunlight.

The onset is gradual and begins with flushing of the cheeks and nose, telangiectasia become noticeable. The condition may then spread to the centre forehead and chin. As the condition progresses, papules, pustules and scales develop. In advanced cases, rhinophyma may occur, the characteristic signs being hypertrophy of the sebaceous glands and thickening of the skin of the nose.

**Table 2.2** Comparison between acne vulgaris and rosacea

| Acne vulgaris | Rosacea |
| --- | --- |
| Develops around the age of puberty, rarely continuing after the age of 30 years | Rarely develops before the age of 30 years |
| Comedones are usually present | Comedones do not occur |
| Sites normally affected: the sides of the face, temples, sides of cheeks, sides of chin, shoulders and front of chest. | Sites affected: the nose, centre cheeks, centre forehead and centre chin. |

**Urticaria**

Urticaria is a condition in which the lesions usually appear rapidly and disappear within minutes or gradually over a number of hours. Other lesions may occur either in the same or in other areas later on. The clinical signs of urticaria are the development of red wheals, which may later become white. The area becomes itchy or may sting, e.g. after touching stinging nettles.

There are numerous causes of urticaria some of which are an allergic reaction to certain foods, e.g. strawberries and shellfish; drugs such as penicillin or aspirin; inhalants such as house dust, animal fur and pollens. Other causes include stress, dermagraphic skin, sensitivity to light, heat or cold.

**Pigmentation disorders**

Some conditions are due either to excess pigmentation or to lack of pigmentation in the skin. These include vitiligo, lentigo and chloasma. Generalized pigmentation may be associated with a systemic disease such as pituitary tumour or Addison's disease.

*Vitiligo* is the name used to describe lack of pigmentation in the skin. Any area can be affected and the size of patches, which may be oval or irregular in shape, can vary from quite small to covering extensive areas. It is most commonly seen on the face and hands. Both sexes of any age group can be affected. The cause is unknown. Patches lacking pigmentation are very sensitive to sunlight, and burn easily.

*Lentigo* is the technical term given to freckles. They tend to appear after exposure to sunlight, and fade during the winter months. They are most commonly seen on red-haired and fair-skinned people.

*Chloasma* is patches of increased pigmentation usually seen on the face during pregnancy. The oral contraceptive pill may also give rise to chloasma. This type of pigmentation usually fades after the pregnancy has ended. It may also occur during the menopause.

*Hyper-pigmentation* is due to sensitization of the skin on exposure to sunlight. Substances such as perfume, certain cosmetic preparations, and citrus-based essential oils, e.g. bergamot, all react with sunlight to produce increased pigmentation. This type of pigmentation, which is known as Berloque dermatitis, may take years to fade.

**Naevi and benign tumours**

There are a number of different naevi, some of which can be easily identified while others cannot. Some naevi may respond to cauterization, some are best left alone and others benefit from medical treatment. With any naevus which may be suitable for cauterization electrolysists should not take it upon themselves to make the final decision but should refer clients back to their general practitioner for written agreement prior to treatment.

*Pigmented naevi*

These may also be referred to as moles. They appear as flat or raised, round, smooth lumps on the surface of the skin. They vary in size and in colour, from pink to brown or black. It is very rare for this type of lesion to become malignant. They are caused by changes in the melanocytes which give rise to cells called 'naevus cells'.

*Port-wine stain*

This is also known as deep capillary naevus, or mature haemangiomata, and is due to an accumulation of dilated capillaries in the dermis and deeper layers of the skin. It is present at birth and may vary in colour from pale pink to deep purple. It has an irregular shape and is not raised above the skin's surface. These naevi are often found on the face but may also appear on other areas of the body.

**Haemangiomata**  These appear as a small, raised, red papule which bleed easily. The cause is unknown but they often appear after vigorous squeezing of skin lesions such as a comedone or papule. They are easily removed by shortwave diathermy.

**Spider naevus**  This refers to a collection of telangiectasia which radiate from a centre papule. They often appear during pregnancy and if left untreated will disappear on their own. Alternatively they are easily dealt with by short-wave diathermy. When multiple naevi are present a liver disease may be indicated.

**Keloid**  This is the term used for an overgrowth of scar tissue. The surface may be smooth and shiny, or ridged. Keloid scars usually appear over the seat of a previous lesion or after surgery along the site of the incision. The onset is gradual and is due to an accumulation or increase of collagen in the immediate area. The colour varies from red, fading to pink or white. There is a racial predisposition to the development of keloids, and they are very common in Negroid skin.

**Fibroma**  These are hard, painless nodules which may be shiny or firm. They are normally found on the extremities.

**Seborrhoeic warts**  Also referred to as senile warts, these are not caused by a viral infection and are not related in any way to other forms of wart. They tend to develop after the age of 40 years. They are normally found on the trunk but may also appear on the face or other areas. Clinical signs indicate hyperkeratosis with increased pigmentation which varies from one lesion to another. The surface is rough and uneven.

**Malignant tumours**
**Malignant melanoma**  This is a rare tumour which develops from a pigmented naevus. Its main characteristic is a blue black nodule which increases in size, shape and colour. These tumours are most commonly found on the head, neck and trunk. Development of this tumour may be either slow or rapid. It should be emphasized that when a mole or tumour shows any change in shape, size or colour, or begins to itch, a doctor should be consulted.

**Basal cell carcinoma**  This is also referred to as basal cell epithelioma or more commonly rodent ulcer. Clinical characteristics of a rodent ulcer are a raised, nodular, shiny lesion with a pearly edge. The surface may become ulcerated. The lesions bleed easily especially when the surface crust is removed. This particular carcinoma most commonly appears on the face and forehead but is not unknown on the arms, legs or trunk. It is caused by excessive exposure of the skin to the sun and is the most common form of skin cancer.

*Squamous cell carcinoma*

This is entirely different from the basal cell carcinoma. It is most frequently seen in elderly people. The onset is gradual. Clinical signs are the presence of a warty surface with ulcerations occurring when the growth is 1 to 2 cm in diameter. The edge of the ulcer thickens. It is a true invasive tumour which develops in normal tissue or in a pre-existing lesion.

## Conclusion

There are very many skin diseases and disorders that professional electrolysists may come into contact with during the course of their work. It will be possible to treat some conditions with electrical epilation, whereas others may be contra-indicated, and a number may indicate referral to the medical profession. It is essential that every electrolysist becomes familiar with the most common conditions and is able to decide which course of action will give most benefit to the client.

## Review questions

1  Name the internal and external influences which affect the health and condition of the skin.
2  Define the term 'skin lesion'.
3  Describe the following:
   (a)  macule;
   (b)  pustule;
   (c)  plaque;
   (d)  vesicle;
   (e)  fissure.
4  Explain the meaning of the term 'hyperkeratosis'.
5  What is the difference between hyper pigmentation and hypo-pigmentation?
6  Name six causes of skin disease.
7  Briefly describe the appearance of:
   (a)  impetigo;
   (b)  herpes zoster;
   (c)  pityriasis versicolor.
8  Name the cause and describe the development of scabies.
9  Define the terms 'eczema' and 'dermatitis'.
10  Describe the appearance of 'allergic dermatitis'.
11  What is the difference between contact dermatitis and allergic dermatitis?
12  Describe the clinical signs of psoriasis and name the aggravating factors.
13  Compare acne vulgaris with rosacea.
14  Give the characteristics of a pigmented naevus.
15  What is a keloid?
16  Give the clinical characteristics of a rodent ulcer.

# 3 Hair

Hair has made its presence felt for thousands of years. For many it is their crowning glory whereas for others it causes much unhappiness and embarrassment, either through growth where it is not required or from loss where it *is* required. Women spend a fortune removing hair by waxing, shaving, depilatory creams or electrical epilation. Many men on the other hand try every remedy that hints of a promise to restore their failing locks.

In order to eliminate hair permanently it is essential to be familiar with its structure and growth cycle.

Hairs are keratinized structures growing out of hair follicles which are sac-like indentations of the epidermis. Keratin is a hard, horny substance which resists digestion by pepsin and is insoluble in water, organic substances, dilute acids and alkali. Organic substances dilute acids and alkalis. Keratin is made up of the elements carbon, hydrogen, sulphur, oxygen and nitrogen.

The hair can be divided into:

1  the shaft – this is the portion above the skin's surface;
2  the root – the portion of hair lying in the follicle;
3  the bulb – the enlarged base of the root, surrounding the papilla.

## Types of hair

Three distinct types of hair are to be found on the human body.

1  lanugo;
2  vellus;
3  terminal.

*Lanugo hair* is usually found in foetal life and is normally shed around the seventh to eighth month of pregnancy. This type of hair is fine, soft, without a medulla and usually unpigmented.

*Vellus hair* is fine, downy, soft and unpigmented. It is found on the body generally, and rarely exceeds 2 cms in length. These hairs do not contain a medulla. The base of the vellus hair lies very close to the skin's surface.

*Terminal hairs* replace vellus hairs at specific sites of the body. They are longer, coarser, pigmented, and varying in shape, diameter, texture, length and colour. They can be divided into asexual, ambisexual and sexual hair.

*Asexual* hair is genetic hair present at birth. This hair type is influenced by changes in growth hormone production but is not dependent on steroid hormones. Asexual hair refers to terminal hair found on the scalp, eyebrows, eyelashes and to a lesser extent on the forearms and legs in both sexes of all ages.

*Ambisexual* hair develops in both sexes at puberty. This type of hair growth is influenced by the increased adrenal and gonadal androgen production. Ambisexual hair is found in the axilla, pubis, lower limbs and abdomen from puberty in both sexes. Growth on the forearms and legs becomes more profuse at this stage of life. The density and rate of hair growth differs widely between the sexes, between individuals of the same sex and between various body sites.

*Sexual hair* includes the beard, moustache, nasal passages, ears and external body hairs, e.g. back and chest. Sexual hair is influenced by increased androgen hormone production by the gonads. Testosterone levels in men are 15–30 per cent higher than in women. Sexual hair is more pronounced in men due to the higher levels of progesterone production by the testes.

The shape of the hair is determined by the shape of the follicle, i.e. straight hairs grow from straight follicles whereas wavy or curly hairs grow from curved follicles. Hairs which are kinked or frizzy grow from follicles which have become distorted at the base due to mechanical interference such as waxing or tweezing.

## Structure of the hair

Terminal hair is composed of three layers (see Figure 3.1):

1  cuticle;
2  cortex;
3  medulla.

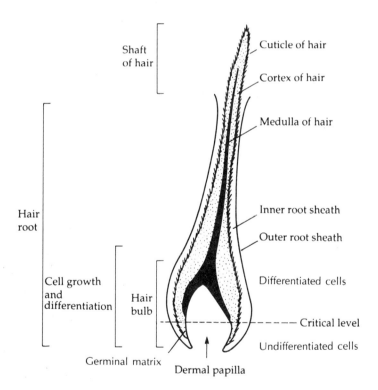

**Figure 3.1** Longitudinal diagram of terminal hair

The *cuticle* consists of a single layer of scale-like cells which point towards the tip of the hair. These cells overlap rather like the tiles on a roof. This overlapping allows the cuticle of the hair to interlock with the cuticle of the hair follicle, so holding the hair in place. A thin layer of lipids (fatty substances) and carbohydrate surrounds the cuticle and may protect the hair from the effects of physical and chemical agents. No pigment is contained in this layer. The function of the cuticle is to confine and protect the cortex and give the hair its elasticity.

The *cortex* lies inside the cuticle and forms the bulk of the hair. It consists of elongated keratinized cells cemented together. Melanin granules are contained within this layer which gives the hair its pigment. A number of air spaces are contained within the cortex. In the living part of the hair these spaces are filled with fluid, which gradually dries out as the hair grows. They are larger at the base of the hair, becoming smaller towards the tip.

The *medulla,* when present, is found in the centre of the hair. It may be continuous or discontinuous and may vary within the same hair. The medulla is formed of loosely connected, keratinized cells. Air spaces in the medulla determine the sheen and colour tones due to the reflection of light.

**The hair follicle**

The hair follicle is a downward extension of the epidermis of the skin. Hair follicles, together with the sebaceous gland, form the pilo-sebaceous system. Attached to the follicle below the sebaceous gland is the arrector pili muscle. It is the contraction of this muscle which causes the hair to stand on end – so giving the goose-pimple effect.

*Structure of the hair follicle*

The hair follicle consists of the following structures:

1 inner root sheath;
2 outer root sheath;
3 vitreous membrane;
4 connective tissue.

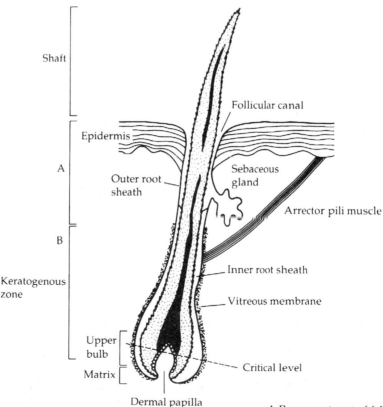

**Figure 3.2** Anagen hair in its follicle

A Permanent part of follicle
B Transient part of hair follicle

The *inner root sheath* holds the hair in the follicle by interlocking with the cuticle of the hair to the level of the sebaceous gland. The inner root sheath is composed of three distinct layers.

1  The innermost layer is the cuticle which interlocks with the cuticle of the hair.
2  Huxley's layer is the middle layer and is the thickest of the three layers.
3  Henle's layer is the outer layer and consists of a single layer of cells.

The inner root sheath originates from the base of the follicle, growing up in unison with the hair until it reaches the level of the sebaceous gland. The hair then continues to grow up, on its own, through the (follicular) hair canal.

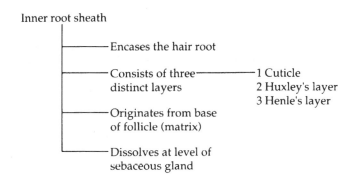

Inner root sheath

— Encases the hair root

— Consists of three ——— 1 Cuticle
distinct layers          2 Huxley's layer
                         3 Henle's layer

— Originates from base
of follicle (matrix)

— Dissolves at level of
sebaceous gland

**Figure 3.3**  The inner root sheath

The *outer root sheath* surrounds the inner root sheath, and is a continuation of the mitotic layer of the epidermis. At the level of the sebaceous gland the cellular structure of this layer cannot be distinguished from that of the surface epidermis. Large amounts of water and glycogen are contained in this layer, the highest concentration being found in the cells between the neck of the bulb up to the level of the sebaceous gland. The thickness of the outer root sheath is uneven. Unlike the inner root sheath it does not grow up in unison with the hair. The outer root sheath is the permanent source of the *hair germ cells* from which new follicles develop when stimulated by circulating hormones and enzymes.

*The hair bulb*

The hair bulb can be divided into upper and lower regions. The lower region contains undifferentiated cells, whereas the cells in the upper region differentiate to form the hair and inner root sheath.

An imaginary line drawn across the widest part of the hair bulb would separate the two regions and is known as the critical level. Below the critical level is the germinative centre or matrix, where all the cells are mitotically active. From the matrix, cells move to the upper part of the bulb where they elongate vertically and increase in volume.

The keratogenous zone is found in the topmost part of the bulb, above the critical level, terminating approximately one-third of the way between the tip of the papilla and the skin's surface. Melanocytes are contained

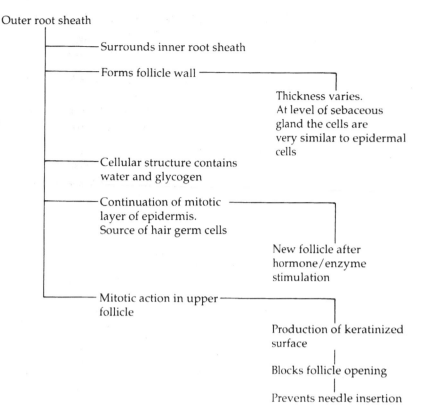

Outer root sheath

— Surrounds inner root sheath

— Forms follicle wall —— Thickness varies. At level of sebaceous gland the cells are very similar to epidermal cells

— Cellular structure contains water and glycogen

— Continuation of mitotic layer of epidermis. Source of hair germ cells —— New follicle after hormone/enzyme stimulation

— Mitotic action in upper follicle —— Production of keratinized surface

Blocks follicle opening

Prevents needle insertion

**Figure 3.4** The outer root sheath

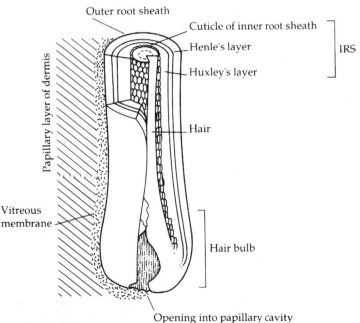

Outer root sheath

Cuticle of inner root sheath ⎤
Henle's layer        ⎥ IRS
Huxley's layer       ⎦

Papillary layer of dermis

Hair

Vitreous membrane

Hair bulb

**Figure 3.5** The bulb of the follicle

Opening into papillary cavity

within the upper part of the bulb and are concerned with pigmentation of the hair. The matrix contains very little melanin, therefore showing the separation of the upper from the lower bulb quite clearly.

The upper bulb can be compared to the spinous layer of the epidermis. In both places indifferent epidermal cells become larger, acquire pigment, synthesize fibrous proteins, become reoriented and undergo the final stages of keratinization. About halfway up the follicle is the keratogenous zone where keratinization takes place.

## The connective tissue sheath

The connective tissue surrounds the outside of the follicle and the sebaceous gland. It is a continuous extension of the papillary layer of the dermis and includes the dermal papilla. The dermal papilla is the main source of sustenance for the entire follicle structure. The vitreous membrane, which is a hyaline, non-cellular glossy membrane, lies next to the outer root sheath. Surrounding the vitreous membrane are two layers of connective tissue. The first layer consists of compact fibres arranged circularly around the follicle. The second layer is composed of longitudinal bundles of connective tissue, which is attached at the base of the follicle to the dermal papilla by a stalk.

## The nerve supply to the follicle

The nerve supply to the skin is contained within the dermis and around the hair follicles, reaching the base of the epidermis. It is this dermal network of nerves to the hair and follicle which forms the skin's sensory nerve supply. The nerve plexus surrounds the hair follicle extending to the upper part of the pilary canal with a few fibres reaching the sebaceous glands. During telogen the follicle is shorter, therefore the nerve supply will be closer to its base.

Tactile stimuli increase the range of sensitivity to minute mechanical disturbances, due to the sensory nerves of the hair follicle.

## Blood supply to the hair follicle

Hair follicles are surrounded by a network of capillaries, the density of which differs between active and resting follicles. The entire follicle, together with the sebaceous gland, is surrounded by this network of capillaries. A loosely woven network of capillaries is formed above the level of the sebaceous gland. This network extends to, and is continuous with, the loops of capillaries found in the *papillary plexus.*

These loops of capillaries form a vascular ring around the terminal part of the pilary canal. In the *dermal papilla* capillaries from a central tuft of vessels extend to the walls of the inner surface of the follicle and practically come into contact with it. The vascular system of each follicle, including the plexus around the sebaceous glands, is a continuous unit (Montagna and Ellis, *Structure and Function of the Skin*).

The vascular system becomes smaller in proportion to the size of the follicle. The lower part of the follicle containing vellus hair has very few capillaries, with no vessels penetrating the dermal papilla.

A number of changes take place during *catagen.* While the vascular system around the bulb and dermal papilla remains intact during early catagen, the vitreous membrane and connective tissue sheath becomes thicker and wrinkled. When the outer root sheath and bulb collapse during late catagen, the blood vessels of the lower plexus remain intact.

When the follicle shortens, the papillary vessels retreat upwards and the vessels of the papilla lose their clear outline.

Some capillary tufts in the dermal papilla collapse and show the first sign of degenerative changes in the vascular system of the follicle.

In advance catagen the lower third of the follicle shrivels, retreating upward, leaving a trail of connective tissue behind known as the *epidermal cord.*

The dermal papilla, freed from the bulb, remains in contact with the retreating follicle via the epidermal cord.

All these changes take place inside the lower vascular network of the follicle, which remains relatively intact even in advanced changes. Some of the capillaries of the lower network degenerate when the lower third of the follicle is reduced to a thin, long strand of cells. At completion of catagen most of the follicle below the bulge is reduced to a hair germ, at the base of which the dermal papilla is attached.

Around the sebaceous gland and funnel-shaped entrance (infundibulum) of the pilary canal, the upper follicular network remains intact and is similar to that around the active follicles. When the resting follicle becomes active again, the new bulb must advance through the collapsed bundle below the dermal papilla, growing inside it. The major vessels of the follicle remain intact during catagenic changes.

Exchange of nutrients takes place through the wall of the bulb that faces the dermal papilla. Not all dermal papillae are equally supplied with vessels, and the amount of vascular tissue in a papilla is related to the size of the follicle. The wider the diameter of the follicle, the larger the capillary tufts it contains. The dermal papillae of active, large human follicles are very wide and contain large numbers of capillaries.

# Hair growth cycle

The follicle goes through three distinct stages of development. These stages are known as anagen, catagen and telogen (see Figure 3.6). Detailed knowledge of the hair growth cycle can be attributed to a number of people, in particular Dry, 1926, Ligman, 1959, Montagna and Parakkal, 1974.

*Anagen* is the active stage which results in the complete restructuring of the lower follicle. Hair germ cells contained within the dermal cord begin to multiply by mitosis. The dermal cord grows downwards into the dermis, at the same time growing in width, until the dermal papilla is engulfed by the bulb which has formed at the tip of the dermal cord.

The specialized nature of papilla cells is maintained even when papillae are isolated from epidermal cells. It has been shown (Orfanos, Montagna and Stuttgen, 1981) that when direct papilla/epidermal contact is maintained the papilla induces the following changes: the development of a matrix; increased mitotic activity of the epidermis; and hair growth and follicle lengthening.

Before the follicle has reached its full depth the mitotic cells of the *germinal* matrix, found in the lower part of the bulb, become active. These cells move upwards differentiating into cells that produce (a) the hair and (b) the inner root sheath.

Towards the end of anagen, thinning and lightening of the pigment at the base of the hair shaft takes place, and melanin production stops. Melanocytes reabsorb their dendrites (Kingman, 1959; Montagna and Parakkal, 1974). During anagen the follicle receives its nourishment through the dermal papilla.

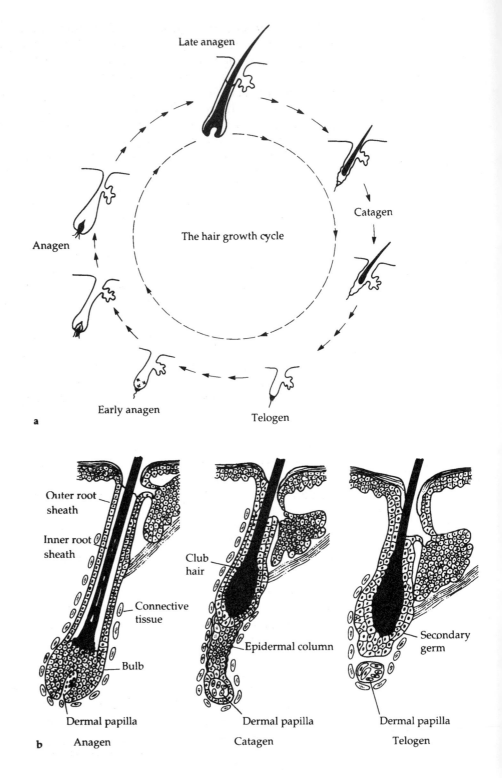

**Figure 3.6** The hair growth cycle

*Catagen* follows on from anagen, this stage being known as the transitional stage where the club hair is formed. The dermal papilla *separates* from the matrix and the hair starts to rise in the follicle. At this time the hair is held in the follicle by the cells of the inner root sheath and receives its nourishment from the follicle wall. As the follicle begins to shrink and collapse below the rising hair, the epidermal cord is formed from undifferentiated cells. The hair becomes drier, losing water and glycogen.

*Telogen* follows on from catagen and is the final phase of the growth cycle. This is known as the quiescent or resting period, when the follicle remains inactive or dormant until stimulated into anagen where the whole process is repeated. Telogen lasts for only a few weeks, with the club hair often being retained within the follicle until the new hair is produced and pushes the club hair out of the follicle. The telogen follicle is one-third to half the length of a full anagen follicle.

To summarize, the hair is a keratinized structure consisting of three layers – cuticle, cortex and medulla – which grows from the hair follicle. The follicle forms part of the pilo-sebaceous unit, which reaches from the epidermis down to the dermal papilla situated in the dermis. The hair follicle goes through a growth cycle divided into three phases, these being anagen – active, catagen – transitional, and telogen – resting. The follicle structure consists of inner and outer root sheaths, the outer root sheath being separated from the connective tissue by a vitreous membrane. Both the follicle and hair receive nourishment from the dermal papilla. Development and growth are stimulated by circulating hormones and enzymes within the blood.

## Glossary

**Hair**   Keratinized structure which grows out of the hair follicle.

**Hair follicle**   Sac-like indentation of the epidermis which grows down to the subjacent dermis.

**Asexual hair**   Growth not governed by hormones, e.g. scalp, eyebrows, eyelashes.

**Sexual hair**   Growth and development influenced by hormones, particularly androgens. Found in the axilla and pubis.

**Pilo-sebaceous unit**   Formed from the hair follicle and the sebaceous gland.

**Hair germ**   Consists of undifferentiated cells, which produce new hair when stimulated by circulating hormones and enzyme action.

**Epidermal cord**   Slender cord of hair germ cells which enables the retreating follicle to maintain contact with the dermal papilla.

**Keratin**   Hard, horny substance made up of carbon, hydrogen, sulphur, oxygen and nitrogen.

**Keratogenous zone**   Area where keratinization takes place in the hair follicle. This is found in the upper part of the bulb and finishes approximately one-third of the way between the tip of the papilla and the skin's surface.

**Anagen**   Active stage of growth where lower follicle rebuilds and new hair is formed.

**Catagen**   Follows anagen. Hair separates from dermal papilla. Club hair is formed. Lower follicle begins to shrivel and collapse.

**Telogen** Final stage of hair growth cycle. Follows catagen. Follicle is inactive or resting and a half to one-third the length of the anagen follicle.
**Club hair** Develops in catagen. The bulb of the hair dries out and becomes brush-like. The club hair is held in the follicle by the cells of the inner root sheath.
**Infundibulum** Funnel-shaped opening to follicle.
**Pilary canal** Consists of upper third portion of the outer root sheath, which extends above the entrance of the sebaceous gland.

## Review questions

1 What is a hair follicle?
2 Draw and label a diagram of a terminal hair in its follicle.
3 Name the structures of an anagen follicle.
4 What is the dermal cord?
5 How does the dermal papilla maintain contact with the follicle?
6 Describe the following: outer root sheath, inner root sheath, hair bulb, connective tissue, vitreous membrane.
7 Name the three stages of the hair growth cycle.
8 Describe the three stages of follicle development and hair growth.
9 What is the function of the arrector pili muscle?
10 What is meant by the 'critical level'?
11 Where is the pigment of the hair to be found?
12 Explain the difference between a vellus and a terminal hair.
13 Describe in detail the structure of a terminal hair.
14 How does the hair receive its nutrients?
15 Define 'keratogenous zone'.
16 What is the function of the germinal matrix?

# 4 Cardiovascular system

It is not the author's intention to cover the cardiovascular system in any depth in this text – there are many good anatomy and physiology books which deal with the subject well. The aim is to give a general insight into the functions and clotting mechanism of blood, so that the electrolysist will understand the role of the cardiovascular system in relation to the following:

- healthy skin and hair
- the endocrine system
- the clotting mechanism at the site of an injury or during the treatment of naevi and capillaries arising out of accidental misprobe.

The human body is composed of a number of organized systems, none of which can function independently. The cardiovascular system acts as the transport medium carrying oxygen, nutrients and hormones etc. to tissue cells while at the same time removing waste products and carbon dioxide via the blood.

Blood is carried through the system via a series of arteries, arterioles, capillaries, venules and veins, with the heart being the receiving and distribution centre (see Figure 4.1).

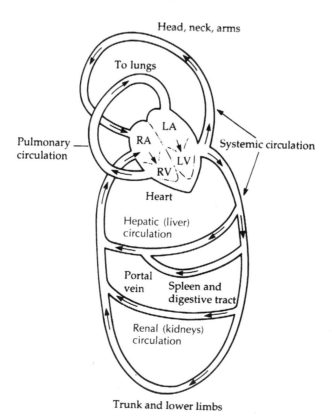

**Figure 4.1** General circulation

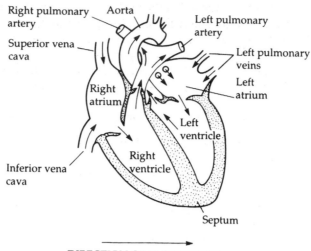

**Figure 4.2** The heart and associated blood vessels

DIRECTION OF BLOOD FLOW

**The heart**

This is a strong, muscular pump which works continuously throughout life. It is made up of four chambers, which are divided into two upper chambers or atrium and two lower chambers or ventricles. The right and left side of the heart is separated by the septum (see Figure 4.2).

The right side of the heart receives dark red deoxygenated blood from the veins. This blood is then transported via the pulmonary artery to the lungs. The left side of the heart receives bright red oxygenated blood from the lungs via the pulmonary vein. This blood leaves the heart through the aorta and passes into the arteries for distribution round the body.

**Arteries**

These are strong, muscular tubes which carry oxygenated blood, hormones, nutrients and other substances to the capillary networks for distribution to the tissue cells. The exception to this rule is the pulmonary artery. Arteries divide into branches called arterioles which in turn divide into smaller capillaries.

**Capillaries**

These form the capillary network where exchange of gases, nutrients, hormones and metabolic waste takes place. The capillary network forms the link between arterioles and venules.

**Venules**

These are the small branches which join up to connect with the veins.

**Veins**

Veins return blood containing carbon dioxide and waste products to the heart for distribution to the lungs. Veins are thinner than arteries. They are not as muscular and contain valves to prevent the backward flow of blood.

**Composition of blood**

Blood is a salty-tasting fluid consisting of plasma and solids. Plasma is an alkaline, straw-coloured substance composed of 91 per cent water, 8 per cent protein and 0.9 per cent salts.

The solids consist of:

1 platelets or thrombocytes which play a part in the control of bleeding after an injury and the clotting procedure;
2 erythrocytes or red cells carrying haemoglobin which combine with oxygen to form oxyhaemoglobin;
3 leucocytes or white cells, their function is to ingest bacteria and protect the body against micro-organisms, thereby fighting infection.

## Function of blood

The function of blood is to act as a transport medium for the following:

- nutrients, tissue salts and enzymes } to tissue cells
- oxygen
- hormones from the endocrine glands to the target organs
- urea
- uric acid } from the cells to the elimination organs
- carbon dioxide
- antibodies to fight infection
- drugs and medication.

Blood is also concerned with temperature control of the body. This is achieved by the vasodilation and vasoconstriction of surface capillaries. When too much heat is present the capillaries dilate to release heat to the surface. When the body is cold the surface capillaries constrict to contain the heat.

Platelets, together with other substances within the blood, are responsible for removing bacteria and micro-organisms from the blood, thereby helping to fight infection. When a foreign body such as an epilation needle or microlance pierces the skin the tip penetrates the surface allowing germs and bacteria to enter the blood stream. Blood brings white cells to the area, their function being to kill the bacteria and germs.

The site of the injury becomes red, swollen, painful and hot due to the increased local blood supply and the activity of the cells in the area. This particular injury is known as 'needle stick injury'. It is possible to transmit hepatitis B and AIDS in this manner if contaminated needles are used.

## Blood clotting mechanism

It is well known that if the skin is cut, grazed or punctured in any way blood will appear at the surface. After a short period of time a clot should form at the area, sealing the skin. Eventually the clot will dry into a scab, which will fall off when the skin underneath has healed. The exception to this is the condition of haemophilia, where clotting does not take place. A severe case of this could lead to the death of the person concerned.

The clotting process relies on a number of factors, as shown in Figure 4.3.

The health and efficiency of the blood vascular system can be affected by:

1 badly balanced or incorrect nutrition;
2 smoking;
3 anti-coagulant drugs such as warfarin and aspirin;
4 alcohol.

When the blood is not able to do its job efficiently the healing rate of the skin after electro-epilation will not be good.

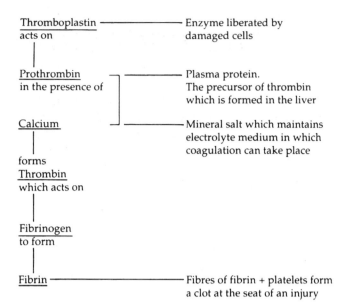

**Figure 4.3** Factors necessary to the clotting process

In clients who smoke regularly, or who perhaps take an aspirin immediately before the treatment of spider naevi or telangiectasia, the blood will not coagulate well.

Clients who follow a badly balanced diet which lacks sufficient nutrients and vitamins, or who eat irregularly, may find that the skin is not as healthy and therefore takes longer to heal after treatment. Frequent quantities of hot, spicy foods, large quantities of strong hot tea or coffee, high quantities of alcohol, and bolting food all aggravate and may weaken the surface capillaries.

## Review questions

1 Draw and label a diagram of the heart.
2 Describe the differences between arteries and veins.
3 What is the composition of blood?
4 What is meant by the blood clotting mechanism?
5 Name four factors which affect the health and efficiency of the blood vascular system.

# 5 The endocrine system

The endocrine system can be referred to as the 'orchestra' of the body, with the conductor being the pituitary gland in conjunction with the hypothalamus, which forms a link between the endocrine and nervous systems. When this system is working in harmony the balance of hormone levels will be correct. This in turn will enable all the other systems of the body to carry out their functions effectively. Body growth, development and functioning are all dependent on the efficiency of the endocrine system. Too much or too little of any hormone will cause an imbalance which will result in certain disorders or malfunction.

The process involved in the endocrine system is shown in Figure 5.1.

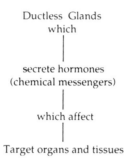

Ductless Glands
which

secrete hormones
(chemical messengers)

which affect

Target organs and tissues

**Figure 5.1** The endocrine system

## Hormones

Hormones are complex chemical substances produced by endocrine glands. Their function is to stimulate or inhibit the action of specific glands, organs or tissues. Hormones are released directly into the bloodstream. They are slow-acting chemical messengers which control functions such as metabolism, growth of body tissues and cells, also mental and physical coordination.

The hypothalamus, pituitary and target glands control the hormone levels in the blood by means of the feedback mechanism. When the level of a particular hormone falls the hypothalamus notifies the pituitary gland to increase secretion of the trophic hormone in order to stimulate hormone production by the target gland, e.g. low levels of thyroxine trigger the hypothalamus into informing the pituitary of the need to increase its output of thyroid stimulating hormone (TSH) which will then influence the thyroid gland to increase secretion of thyroxine. In reverse when there is a high level of a particular hormone the hypothalamus will inform the pituitary to decrease secretion of the trophic hormone (see Figure 5.2).

Without the correct balance of hormones it is not possible to lead a healthy life. Stress control, metabolism, body growth, sexual development, temperature regulation and memory are some of the functions which are dependent on the presence of hormones.

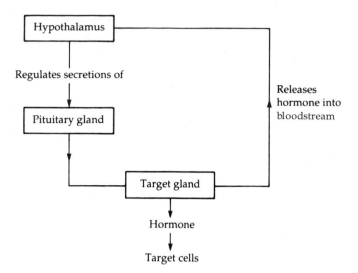

**Figure 5.2** The feedback mechanism

# Endocrine glands

The endocrine glands are situated in specific sites of the body. They are ductless glands which produce *hormones*, secreting them directly into the bloodstream. These glands of internal secretion work closely with the nervous system to form the communication network of the body (see Figure 5.3).

The glands differ in shape, size and location although their function is the same, i.e. to produce hormones.

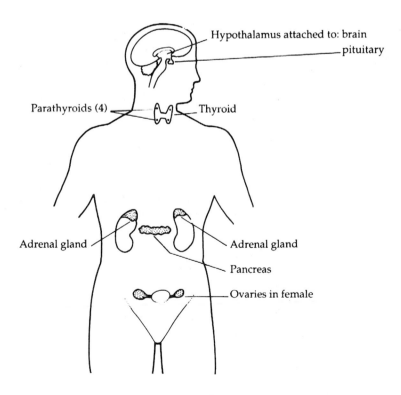

**Figure 5.3** Positions of the endocrine glands

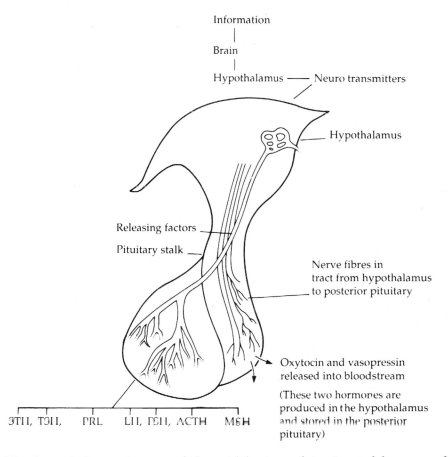

Information
|
Brain
|
Hypothalamus —— Neuro transmitters

Hypothalamus

Releasing factors

Pituitary stalk

Nerve fibres in
tract from hypothalamus
to posterior pituitary

Oxytocin and vasopressin
released into bloodstream

(These two hormones are
produced in the hypothalamus
and stored in the posterior
pituitary)

GTH, TSH,    PRL    LH, FSH, ACTH    MSH

**Figure 5.4** The
Hypothalamus

## The
## hypothalamus

The hypothalamus is part of the mid brain and is situated between the thalamus and the pituitary gland. It links the cerebral cortex of the brain with the pituitary by means of a stalk richly supplied with nerve fibres and blood vessels.

The hypothalamus produces releasing and inhibiting hormones which directly affect the pituitary gland. The releasing hormones stimulate the release of trophic hormones into the bloodstream, whereas inhibiting hormones prevent the release of prolactin and melanocyte stimulating hormones. Vasopressin and oxytocin are both produced by the hypothalamus and stored in the posterior pituitary gland.

The role of the hypothalamus is coordination of the endocrine and autonomic nervous systems. It is responsible for the control of:

1   the autonomic nervous system;
2   metabolic processes;
3   secretion of pituitary hormones;
4   sleep;
5   appetite;
6   regulation of sexual function;
7   body temperature;
8   water balance;
9   emotion.

35

Due to the connection with the central nervous system, stress and emotional disturbances may upset the hypothalamic–pituitary mechanism.

## The pituitary gland

The pituitary gland (hypophysis), is known as the 'master gland' of the endocrine system due to its influence on the other endocrine glands.

This gland is situated at the base of the brain in the sella turcica, or pituitary fossa of the sphenoid bone. It is a small round structure in the region of 13 mm in size and weighing approximately 0.6 gs. A small stalk, called the infundibulum, connects the pituitary gland to the hypothalamus.

The pituitary gland is divided into two portions – anterior and posterior – which differ in origin, structure and function. The anterior section is composed of vascular, glandular tissue responsible for the production and secretion of six hormones. The posterior section is composed of nerve-like tissue supplied from the hypothalamus and is responsible for the storage and release of two hormones. Both sections are under hypothalamic control.

### The anterior pituitary gland

The anterior pituitary gland (adenohypophysis) is connected to the hypothalamus by a network of blood vessels through which pass the releasing and inhibiting factors that control pituitary secretion. Pituitary trophic hormones exert their influence on other endocrine glands. Each trophic hormone influences a specific target gland. Hormones produced by the anterior pituitary are as follows:

### 1 Somatotrophic, STH or growth hormone

This controls the growth of bones and formation of tissues. It has an effect on protein, fat and carbohydrate metabolism and promotes the retention of nitrogen.

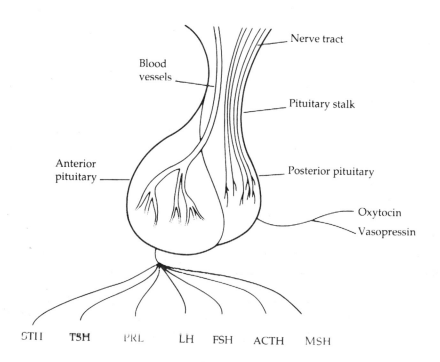

**Figure 5.5** The pituitary gland

Over-secretion of STH leads to pituitary giants in children or enlarged face, hands and feet in adults (acromegaly). Under-secretion in children results in pituitary dwarfs due to under-development of the long bones.

**2 Adreno-corticotrophin (ACTH)**

This controls the adrenal cortex stimulating secretion of steroids. Insufficient stimulation of the adrenal cortex by ACTH results in the gland shrinking. Too much secretion causes enlargement of the gland and an excess production of androgens. Prolonged periods of stress result in increased stimulation of the adrenal gland and therefore higher levels of circulating androgens, which may result in increased hair growth.

**3 Thyroid stimulating hormone (TSH)**

This stimulates the thyroid to produce hormones for regulating body metabolism.

**4 Gonadotrophic hormones**

These stimulate the sex glands and are known as follicle stimulating hormone (FSH) and luteinizing hormone (LH) in the female. LH in the male is known as interstitial cell stimulating hormone.

FSH stimulates the ovarian follicle in the female to ripen and produce oestrogen. In the male the testes are stimulated to produce spermatozoa.

LH in the female stimulates the corpus luteum in the ovary and also secretion of oestrogen and progesterone. In the male the testes are stimulated to produce testosterone. LH influences the development and maintenance of male sex characteristics. In both sexes LH stimulates androgen production by the sex organs.

**5 Prolactin (PRL)**

This is responsible for stimulating milk production from the breasts.

**6 Melanocyte stimulating hormone (MSH)**

This is responsible for stimulation of melanocytes to produce melanin pigment, which results in darkening of the skin.

## The posterior pituitary gland

The posterior pituitary gland stores two hormones which are produced by the hypothalamus. These are oxytocin and vasopressin.

**Oxytocin**

This stimulates contractions of the uterus during labour, and also aids the flow of milk after birth by stimulating lining cells of the breast ducts.

**Vasopressin (ADH)**

This is known as the antidiuretic hormone and is concerned with the maintenance of the body water balance. It influences the renal ducts of the kidneys and water metabolism.

## The thyroid gland

The thyroid gland, the largest endocrine gland, consists of two oval lobes which are situated in the neck just below the larynx, either side and slightly to the front of the trachea. The two lobes are connected by the isthmus, which is a narrow part of the gland (see Figure 5.6).

The thyroid relies on the normal functioning of the pituitary gland for stimulation by TSH to produce three hormones:

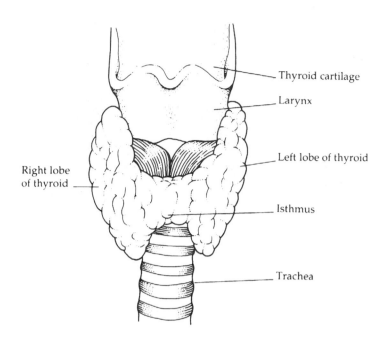

Thyroid cartilage

Larynx

Left lobe of thyroid

Right lobe of thyroid

Isthmus

Trachea

**Figure 5.6** The thyroid gland

1 thyroxine;
2 tri-iodothyronine;
3 calcitonin.

These three hormones control metabolism with thyroxine and tri-iodothyronine, affecting general metabolism and function of the body. Calcitonin affects calcium metabolism. Iodine from food combines with protein to form thyroglobulin which is later changed by the action of enzymes to thyroxine for release into the bloodstream as required.

**Hyperthyroidism (Graves' disease)**

When too much thyroxine is produced a number of problems arise. The person becomes mentally full of energy but is unable to keep up physically. Because of increased metabolism, weight loss occurs. Increased heartbeat, palpitations, profuse sweating, anxiety and heat intolerance are other symptoms associated with over-production of thyroid hormones.

**Hypothyroidism (Myxoedema)**

When insufficient thyroxine is produced the body's metabolism will slow down. The individual may become slow and lethargic, lose concentration easily, feel the cold and experience a steady weight increase. The body temperature is usually subnormal. The skin becomes dry, and hair growth may be sparse, dry and lifeless.

**The parathyroid glands**

The parathyroid glands are four small glands embedded on the back and side surfaces of the thyroid gland. Their role is to produce the hormone parathormone.

Parathormone and calcitonin are responsible for maintaining the calcium levels in the blood. Calcitonin is released when calcium levels are too low. Hair development is affected by calcium levels which when too low will

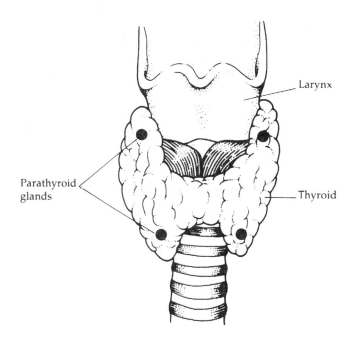

**Figure 5.7** The parathyroid glands

result in sparse, dry brittle hair. High calcium levels can lead to serious bone disorders or kidney stones.

## The pancreas gland

The pancreas is situated in the curve of the duodenum, behind the stomach. This gland has two functions:

1 exocrine – production of pancreatic enzymes to aid digestion in the small intestine;
2 endocrine – production of insulin and glucagon.

Specialized cells known as the islets of Langerhans form the endocrine section and are divided into alpha and beta cells. Alpha cells are responsible for the production of insulin and beta cells for the production of glucagon.

Insulin controls carbohydrate metabolism. Its role is to lower blood sugar levels by promoting entry of sugar into body cells for metabolism or by encouraging glucogen storage in the muscles and liver.

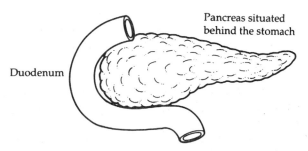

**Figure 5.8** The pancreas

Pancreas tissue contains 1–2 per cent endocrine cells called 'islets of Langerhans'

Glucagon is responsible for raising the blood sugar levels by freeing stored glycogen from the liver.

*Diabetes mellitus* occurs when there is insufficient insulin present in the blood. This disorder affects both sexes but its development is not uncommon during pregnancy and menopause.

Symptoms associated with diabetes mellitus are:

1 increased thirst;
2 increased output of urine;
3 weight loss;
4 thin skin with reduced healing ability;
5 increased tendency to develop minor skin infections;
6 lowered natural body defence against infection;
7 decreased pain threshold when insulin levels are low.

The electrolysist should give careful consideration to the above points when planning treatment sessions for the client who has diabetes (see pages 130 and 135).

## The adrenal glands

The adrenal glands are two triangular-shaped glands which lie in front of and above each kidney. Each gland consists of an outer cortex which is yellow in colour and an inner dark reddish medulla.

The *medulla* is closely linked to the sympathetic nervous system and produces two hormones, adrenalin (epinephrine) and noradrenaline (norepinephrine). The medulla has a complex nerve supply which controls the dilation and contraction of blood vessels. The functions of adrenalin are as follows:

1 stimulates metabolism resulting in the release of glycogen as glucose into the bloodstream thereby raising blood sugar;
2 brings about the contraction of the arterioles in the skin and internal organs;
3 encourages increased oxygen intake by dilating the bronchioles in the lungs;
4 dilates arterioles in the heart and muscles.

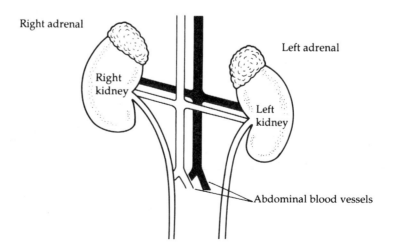

**Figure 5.9** The adrenal glands

Adrenalin is responsible for the activation of the 'fight and flight mechanism' in times of fear, anger or emergency. When this mechanism is activated the muscles receive an increased supply of sugar, blood and oxygen and therefore function more efficiently. The heart-rate is increased. The surface and abdominal blood vessels contract so that the blood supply can be directed to the muscles. Movement of the digestive tract slows down.

Noradrenaline, the second hormone produced by the medulla has an effect on the circulation by contracting blood vessels and raising blood pressure.

The *outer adrenal cortex* produces three groups of hormones:

1  glucocorticoids;
2  mineral corticoids;
3  sex corticoids.

*Glucocorticoids* are concerned with carbohydrate, fat and protein metabolism. This group includes cortisone and hydrocortisone which affect growth of connective tissue.

*Mineral corticoids* which include aldosterone, regulate electrolyte (salt) and water balance in the body.

*Sex corticoids/steroids* act as an auxiliary source of male and female sex hormones. These hormones affect the development and functioning of reproductive organs. They also influence the physical and temperament characteristics in both sexes. When hydrocortisone levels fall the hypothalamus produces more releasing factor so stimulating the pituitary to secrete ACTH in order to restore hydrocortisone production by the adrenal cortex. As a result androgen levels are raised, consequently increasing hair growth in androgen sensitive follicles.

Stress, hyperplasia and adrenal tumours may all bring about excessive steroid secretion, which in turn can stimulate hair growth.

# The ovaries

The ovaries are two small glands which form part of the female reproductive system. They are situated in the pelvic cavity on each side of the uterus and are attached to the fallopian tubes by strong ligaments.

The ovaries have two functions:

1  to produce the hormones oestrogen and progesterone, and small quantities of androgens.
2  to produce ova (eggs).

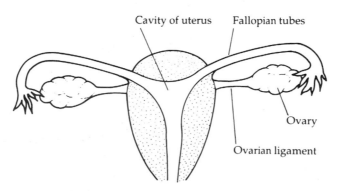

Cavity of uterus    Fallopian tubes

Ovary

Ovarian ligament

**Figure 5.10**  The ovaries

Ovarian hormones become active at puberty and are responsible for development of secondary sex characteristics. Oestrogen is concerned with breast development, growth of the milk ducts in the breast, health and growth of bones, and subcutaneous fat distribution. Oestrogen influences the menstrual cycle and thickens the uterus lining in preparation for conception. It also has an effect on the brain, skin, arteries, veins and muscles. Oestrogen production by the ovaries begins to decline as the menopause approaches. Progesterone is known as the pregnancy hormone. It is concerned with the development of the placenta, maintenance of the pregnancy and also helps to prepare the mammary glands for lactation.

Menstrual disorders occur when the ovary fails to respond to stimulation by the pituitary gonadotrophic hormones, or when there is an abnormal response to stimulation. Increased androgen production by the ovary may give rise to hirsutism.

## The pineal and thymus glands

The pineal and thymus are both endocrine glands, however neither gland has any known influence on hair growth. Recent studies have shown that the pineal has inhibitory and stimulatory influences on the hypothalamus (*The Cause and Management of Hirsutism*, Greenblatt, Mahesh and Gambrell).

The pineal is a small gland situated at the base of the brain. The thymus lies high in the chest.

## Review questions

1  Name the glands which make up the endocrine system.
2  What is a hormone?
3  Describe the role of the hypothalamus.
4  Name and give the functions of the pituitary secretions.
5  What is the role of thyroxine?
6  Describe the two functions of the pancreas.
7  List the symptoms associated with diabetes mellitus.
8  Describe the function of the hormones secreted by the adrenal cortex.
9  What is the fight and flight mechanism?
10  Why is it necessary for the electrolysist to be familiar with the physiology of the endocrine system?

# 6 Hirsutism and hypertrichosis

The terms hirsutism and hypertrichosis are often confused, although there is a definite difference between the two. Both terms are used to describe excessive hair growth in women, but there the similarity ends. Figure 6.1 displays the main features of each.

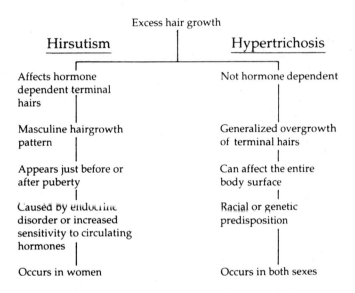

Excess hair growth

| Hirsutism | Hypertrichosis |
|---|---|
| Affects hormone dependent terminal hairs | Not hormone dependent |
| Masculine hairgrowth pattern | Generalized overgrowth of terminal hairs |
| Appears just before or after puberty | Can affect the entire body surface |
| Caused by endocrine disorder or increased sensitivity to circulating hormones | Racial or genetic predisposition |
| Occurs in women | Occurs in both sexes |

**Figure 6.1** Excess hair growth

*Hypertrichosis* is the term used for a generalized overgrowth of vellus and terminal hairs in either sex. Hairs grow longer and faster than normal, although there is no increase in diameter size. This type of hair growth is not due to a systemic disorder. Causes are genetic and racial tendencies, or constitutional variation in follicle sensitivity.

*Hirsutism* refers to a masculine pattern of hair growth in women – one which is normal in men. There is an increase in cyclic growth, diameter of hair and rate of growth. Hirsutism is caused by the following two factors:

1 Increased follicle sensitivity to normal levels of circulating androgens in the bloodstream. This is referred to as primary hirsutism.
2 Increased androgen production by the adrenal glands and ovaries. This is referred to as secondary or true hirsutism. The onset of primary hirsutism occurs at puberty, increasing until the thirties when it stabilizes, whereas secondary hirsutism begins either just before or just after puberty. Secondary hirsutism is due to an endocrine disorder which causes increased hormonal secretion by the glands.

The number and distribution of hair follicles is the same in both sexes. It is genetic predisposition which determines the sex of an individual and specific hair growth patterns. Endocrine hormones are responsible for influencing and stimulating growth at the follicle cells, which in turn determines the pattern, quantity, texture and distribution of body hair.

It is important for clients to understand that both primary and secondary hirsutism can be successfully managed with medical treatment, which will correct or control endocrine disorders thereby preventing the development of new growth. Electrical epilation will eventually remove the existing hair growth permanently. It must be explained to the client that established growth did not appear overnight, and that time is therefore needed to eliminate the problem permanently. The fact that results are slow but sure should be emphasized.

## Causes of hair growth

In order to achieve a successful result with electro-epilation it is necessary for the electrolysist to understand the causes of hair growth. This cannot be fully achieved without first having studied the endocrine system (see Chapter 5).

Consideration should be given to genetic/heredity tendencies, topical causes, and sensitivity of existing follicles to circulating androgens in the bloodstream.

The highest percentage of hirsute women have either a hereditary predisposition or some subtle change in their androgen production.

Hair distribution, type of hair and rate of growth varies from one race to another and from one person to another, for example Caucasians have a higher number of hair follicles than the Japanese and Chinese. Some find the presence of hair both desirable and acceptable whereas others prefer a total absence of hair.

Sensitivity of follicle end receptors to circulating androgens encompasses a number of factors from topical friction to endocrine influences. The degree of hormone sensitivity can vary from one area to another and between different individuals. Increased sensitivity of androgen receptors in the pilo sebaceous unit may be a dominant or recessive hereditary trait.

*Topical causes* include sustained friction such as a plaster cast. Friction causes an increase in local blood circulation to the skin. This type of hair growth is temporary and usually returns to normal shortly after the plaster caste has been removed.

The tweezing of individual hairs tears out the lower follicle. The reconstructed follicle is usually stronger with a better blood supply. Vellus and fine hairs are frequently removed at the same time, so aggravating the condition. Waxing of facial and vellus hair will have the same effect as tweezing. Hairs which have been waxed or tweezed invariably leave behind distorted follicles, so hindering electro-epilation unless blend or galvanic electrolysis is used.

*Endocrine influences* can be divided into normal systemic and abnormal systemic conditions. Normal systemic conditions include: puberty; pregnancy; menopause; stress and sensitivity of follicle end organ receptors to androgens. Abnormal endocrine conditions include: polycystic ovary syndrome – Stein-Leventhal syndrome; Cushings syndrome; adrenal tumours; ovarian tumours; diabetes mellitus; and anorexia nervosa.

Androgens and growth hormones increase the size and diameter of hair growth. Cortisols, oestrogens and thyroid hormones influence and alter without stimulating hair growth. Although oestrogens do not initiate growth they can prolong an existing hair growth cycle. (*The Cause and Management of Hirsutism,* Greenblatt et al.).

*Surgery* can also contribute towards the development of unwanted hair, e.g. a total hysterectomy which involves removal of the ovaries and therefore alters the hormone balance.

# Normal endocrine influences

## Puberty

The anterior pituitary gland secretes gonadotrophic hormones which influence the target organs. These are the ovaries in the female and the testes in the male. At this stage of life the adrenal cortex becomes active. Between them, the adrenal cortex and the gonads secrete large quantities of steroid hormones into the circulatory system.

The appearance of both pubic and axillary hair is due to the increased level of adrenocortical androgens. Hereditary sensitivity in combination with the amount of hormone produced is responsible for the appearance of hair in other areas. Women produce smaller quantities of androgen than men. Androgen levels increase in women during puberty, pregnancy and menopause.

## Pregnancy

During pregnancy there is an increase in hormone activity. On occasions excess androgens are produced with the result that fine hair growth may appear on the lip, chin and sides of the face. Quite often this is a temporary growth which disappears shortly after the end of pregnancy.

## Menopause

The menopause marks the end of a woman's reproductive life. Between the ages of 40 and 50 there is a gradual decline in the oestrogen and progesterone levels due to ovarian tissue slowly ceasing to respond to stimulation by the gonadotrophic hormones of the anterior pituitary gland. Facial hair often develops because of the increased level of circulating androgens.

## Emotional stress

The adrenal glands could be termed the 'stress glands', of the body. They control the fight and flight mechanism. When the body is under stress, either emotionally or physically, the activity of the adrenal glands is increased. During stress the hypothalamus triggers the anterior pituitary gland to produce increased levels of adrenocorticotrophic hormone (ACTH). This in turn stimulates the adrenal glands to produce adrenalin, at the same time increasing androgen production. When stimulation takes place over a prolonged period of time hair growth may occur.

## Medications

Certain medications are known to stimulate or aggravate hair growth. Hormonal medications with androgenic properties may cause hair to grow in a masculine pattern. This type of drug includes testosterone, some oral contraceptives, and anabolic steroids.

# Endocrine disorders which affect hair growth

Endocrine disorders arise out of a glandular defect which may be inherited from either parent or which may be an acquired disease. Disorders which affect hair growth are: Cushings syndrome, Stein-Leventhal syndrome (polycystic ovary syndrome), masculinizing ovarian tumours, adrenogenital syndrome, and adrenal neoplasms.

## Adrenal influences in hirsute women

People vary greatly in their skin sensitivity to androgens due to their genetic background: a high level of circulating androgens may have no effect on one individual, whereas a low level may induce hair growth in another.

### Adrenogenital syndrome

Adrenogenital syndrome fortunately is a rare condition and very unlikely to be seen by the practising electrolysist. The effect of androgen disorder is more noticeable in girls, who show an abnormal development of the external genitalia. In extreme cases the clitoris protrudes and may be mistaken for a penis. The adult female will eventually have a male build and develop a deep voice as well as a male distribution of hair growth.

When a boy is affected he will reach puberty between the ages of three and five years, with secondary sex characteristics becoming noticeable. High androgen levels in both sexes cause rapid body growth which stops early. The epiphyses in the bones fuse at an earlier age than normal.

Symptoms which may be present in the adult woman are due to over-secretion of androgens. These include: receding hairline; the appearance of bald patches; increased hair growth in a masculine pattern on the face and limbs; breasts becoming atrophied, the menstrual cycle may be absent or become irregular. Feminine fat is replaced by masculine muscle.

### Adrenal tumours

These are small non-encapsulated masses, and are usually single solitary nodules. Adrenal tumours (also known as neoplasms) can occur at any age, although they are more common around the age of 30 to 40 years. Their presence is indicated by a sudden onset of virilization or Cushings syndrome. This type of tumour may be masculinizing, causing hirsutism, increased muscle mass and deepening of the voice in women.

### Virilizing congenital adrenal hyperplasias

Virilizing congenital adrenal hyperplasias are the result of enzyme deficiency which affects the production and levels of adrenal hormones. Partial or total enzyme deficiency results in decreased cortisol levels. The brain stimulates the pituitary to release ACTH in order to restore the cortisol levels. At the same time production of androgen is increased by the adrenal cortex, leading to an excess and thereby causing hirsutism.

### Cushings syndrome

Cushings syndrome is brought on by an excess of glucocorticoids as a result of a tumour or excessive adrenal cortex function. Pituitary tumours and certain cancers such as lung and pancreatic cancers result in over-production of ACTH. Increased levels of ACTH lead to an excess of cortisol, androgen and aldosterone production.

There are a number of symptoms associated with Cushings syndrome which include: osteoporosis, due to decreased calcium absorption; obesity of the trunk with purple stretch marks on the abdomen; muscular weakness and wasting of the limbs; skin becomes thin and bruises easily; rounding of the face due to fat deposits in the cheeks; diabetes could occur due to increased steroid production; salt retention leading to high blood pressure and oedema; vellus hair growth due to increased cortisol levels; and excess androgens possibly leading to hirsutism.

**Stein-Leventhal syndrome**

This condition is also known as polycystic ovary syndrome. The electrolysist may be the first person to observe the signs which indicate that a client may be suffering from this condition. Referral of the client back to her doctor for further investigation is advisable. Symptoms associated with polycystic ovary syndrome include: enlarged ovaries with numerous follicular cysts; irregular menstrual cycle; weight gain; and the development of excess hair growth. The onset of hirsutism is gradual, occurring from puberty onwards. Polycystic ovaries are capable of secreting large quantities of androgens.

**Masculinizing ovarian tumours**

This type of tumour is rare, but when present it may cause an excess production of androgen. Hirsutism caused by masculinizing ovarian tumours has a rapid onset, usually but not always in later life. Menstruation may stop and will only start again after surgery.

**Archard-Thiers syndrome**

This is another relatively rare endocrine disorder. The characteristics include: generalized obesity; diabetes mellitus; hypertension; and hirsutism. Hair growth is most noticeable on the face, with emphasis on the moustache and beard. Menstrual disorders may occur.

**Anorexia nervosa**

Anorexia nervosa is a condition which usually affects adolescent girls. It is a condition that involves the nervous, endocrine and digestive systems.

Anorexia nervosa exhibits a number of characteristics which include: an increase in vellus hair growth on the face, trunk and arms; persistent refusal to eat food; absence of menstrual periods; weight loss and wasting muscles; emotional stress or disturbance

Other features associated with this condition are the sufferer's disgust with her personal appearance, a strong conviction that she is overweight and lack of self-esteem. Initially it is possible to keep the problem hidden from other people, but over a period of time a sharp-eyed relative, friend, associate or tutor will become aware of the situation. The anorexic person will persistently refuse to acknowledge that a problem exists.

# Evaluating the cause of hair growth

Before electro-epilation treatment commences the cause of the hair growth should be assessed. It may well be advisable for the client to be referred for medical investigation, after which electro-epilation can begin.

A detailed consultation may give many clues as to the cause of the problem. The hair growth rate and pattern should be looked at. Questions should be asked relating to the onset of the problem. Hair growth which appeared at puberty and has not altered since gives little cause for concern, usually responding well to electro-epilation. A recent onset of hair growth, or one that is getting worse, needs further investigation. Examination of the skin and questions relating to the client's weight may also give valuable clues, for example the presence of acne-type lesions, excessive sebaceous secretion and an increase in weight may be connected to excess androgen production.

# Review questions

1  (a) What is meant by the terms 'hirsutism' and 'hypertrichosis'?
   (b) Compare the two conditions.
2  Explain the role of androgens in hirsutism.

3  Explain how menopause influences hair growth.
4  Explain how emotional stress can stimulate hair growth.
5  What is the cause of virilizing congenital adrenal hyperplasia?
6  Describe the signs and symptoms of Stein-Leventhal syndrome.
7  Name the characteristics and symptoms associated with anorexia nervosa.
8  How does a detailed consultation help when evaluating the cause of hair growth?

# 7 Natural hormone changes which occur during a woman's life

Throughout a woman's reproductive life her hormone balance and levels are constantly changing. From puberty through to menopause the levels of oestrogen and progesterone are never static. The different phases to consider are:

1  puberty;
2  the menstrual cycle;
3  pregnancy;
4  the menopause.

Each relies on the smooth functioning of the feedback mechanism between the hypothalamus, the anterior pituitary and the ovaries. When any one of these three fails to function at 100 per cent efficiency a hormone imbalance will occur which may result in disorders such as endometriosis, polycystic ovaries or menstrual irregularities.

## Puberty

Puberty marks the time of change from childhood to womanhood. Hormone levels start to rise, sex organs become functional and the menstrual cycle begins. Hormonal changes precede physical changes and begin well before the first menstrual period.

Puberty normally begins around the age of 11 years but can vary between the ages of 10 to 15 years. The onset of puberty may be influenced by genetic, endocrine, nutritional, physical and environmental factors.

The process begins when the hypothalamus stimulates the anterior pituitary gland to secrete gonadotrophic hormones which activate the sex glands. The hormones secreted by the anterior pituitary gland at this time are:

1  *adrenocorticotrophic hormone* which stimulates the adrenal cortex to produce oestrogen and progesterone in the female, testosterone and a little oestrogen in the male, also androgens in both sexes;
2  *follicle stimulating hormone* which influences the ovaries to stimulate the maturing Graafian follicles and produce oestrogen.
3  *luteinizing hormone* which stimulates the formation and secretion of the corpus luteum, which in turn secretes progesterone.

## Changes which take place during puberty

Puberty is not an easy time for the young adolescent girl, or for her parents. There are a number of psychological and physical changes. The appearance of acne can affect self-confidence. The individual can become difficult, argumentative, shy or aggressive and may require a great deal of patience.

Initially the menstrual cycle is irregular but usually settles down in time. Fine, dark hair growth may appear on the upper lip and sides of the face due to specific sensitivity to circulating androgens. The rate at which the individual develops in comparison to her contemporaries often causes stress.

Normal changes which take place are as follows:

1 breast development;
2 alteration of body contours due to the laying down of feminine fat deposits, widening of the pelvis, strengthening of the muscles, and change in the shape of the face and jaw;
3 growth of pubic and axillary hair;
4 maturation of the genital tract;
5 increased growth in height and development;
6 emotional and temperament changes;
7 start of menstruation – the average age being 12.8 months;
8 adrenal cortex reaches maturity due to stimulation by the hypothalamus and anterior pituitary gland.

## The menstrual cycle

The normal menstrual cycle starts at puberty and usually finishes during the menopause, with a natural interruption during pregnancy. Conditions such as endocrine disorders, stress, anorexia nervosa and surgery e.g. hysterectomy can alter, suppress or stop the menstrual cycle. The average cycle is 28 days, but cycles can vary between 17 and 42 days (see Figure 7.1). It is the pre-ovulatory phase which varies in length, with the post-ovulatory phase normally lasting 14 days.

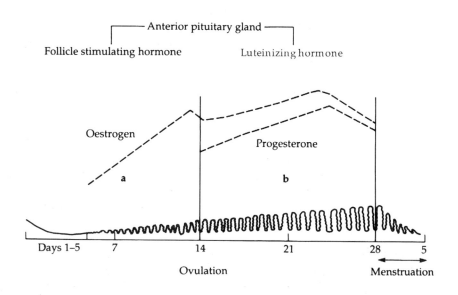

**Figure 7.1** The menstrual cycle

a Proliferation (rebuilding of endometrium) stage is under the influence of oestrogen
b Progesterone influences premenstrual phase

50

The cycle begins when the pituitary gland secretes follicle-stimulating hormone which induces ripening of an ovarian follicle into a mature Graafian follicle. The follicle grows and expands, finally appearing on the ovary surface. Oestrogen, secreted by the growing follicle, thickens the uterus lining (endometrium). Glandular size and richness of blood vessels are increased. After approximately 10 days the pituitary gland secretes luteinizing hormone which in combination with follicle stimulating hormone causes the Graafian follicle to rupture and release an ovum (egg). The egg passes down the Fallopian tube into the uterus, ready for fertilization to take place. The level of follicle stimulating hormone falls at the time of ovulation and remains low for the rest of the cycle.

When the egg breaks free from the ovary it leaves behind a small amount of scar tissue. This tissue develops into the corpus luteum – a yellow gland. For approximately two weeks the corpus luteum produces progesterone in order to enrich the lining membrane of the uterus in preparation for pregnancy. The blood supply to the uterus is increased. When fertilization does not take place after 12 to 14 days the corpus luteum shrinks, progesterone secretion stops, oestrogen levels fall, and blood vessels close and die. Menstruation will then take place: the lining membrane (endometrium) breaks down and is shed in the form of blood, together with the unfertilized egg. Menstruation lasts between three and five days.

## Menstrual cycle ending in pregnancy

When the egg is fertilized by a sperm it becomes implanted into the hormonally-prepared uterus lining. A foetus will then grow. The ordinary ovarian cycle is suspended during pregnancy which usually last nine months from the date of conception.

After fertilization of the egg the corpus luteum continues to grow, reaching its peak after approximately six weeks. The activity of the corpus luteum falls off after approximately two months, finally stopping around the fourth month. The role of the corpus luteum during the early stages of pregnancy is to secrete large amounts of progesterone which is essential for development of the placenta.

The placenta, which develops from the implanted embryo, also produces progesterone, gradually taking this role over from the corpus luteum. The purpose of placental progesterone is to maintain pregnancy and to help prepare the mammary glands for lactation.

Some women notice an increase in excess hair growth during pregnancy, also the appearance of telangiectasia and spider naevi. Often this is temporary and will disappear without treatment shortly after the pregnancy has ended. Telangiectasia which appear on the legs during pregnancy frequently remain, but treatment by shortwave diathermy for these particular capillaries is rarely successful.

## Premenstrual tension

*Premenstrual tension* is the name given to a collection of mental and physical symptoms which occur for up to ten days before menstruation. Symptoms include fluid retention, temporary weight gain, distended abdomen, swollen ankles, breasts becoming tender, irritability and temperament changes. Accidents and clumsiness are common at this time. Pain threshold is lower, therefore the individual is often more sensitive to current intensity during electro-epilation. Hair growth appears to be faster immediately prior to menstruation. The cause of these symptoms is believed to be an imbalance between oestrogen and progesterone.

## The menopause

It is possible that a woman will live a third of her life after the menopause. The menopause is the time when a woman's reproductive function comes to an end. Menstruation becomes irregular and finally stops. The ovaries' supply of fertile eggs dries up. There is a decline in hormone production by the ovaries from the age of 40 onwards, with the menopause usually occurring between the ages of 45 and 55. Some 90 per cent of women stop their periods between the ages of 45 and 55 years. As the level of oestrogen decreases, the amount of free testosterone increases.

A premature menopause will be brought about by surgical removal of the ovaries and womb, in other words a total hysterectomy.

There are a number of symptoms a woman may experience when she reaches the menopause. Unwanted hair growth may appear due to the lowering of the oestrogen levels and follicle sensitivity to circulating androgens. There may be varying degrees of vasomotor instability, giving rise to hot flushes and night sweats. Depression, headaches, bladder irritations, vaginal dryness, painful intercourse, cystitis, insomnia, loss of confidence, poor concentration, tiredness as well as demineralization of bones (osteoporosis) and aching joints can all occur during this period of life.

Intermediate symptoms are dry hair and skin, dryness of the vagina, loss of libido, and bladder infections. Long-term loss of oestrogen may result in osteoporosis, heart attacks or strokes. Oestrogen has been found to reduce heart attacks by 50 per cent and strokes by 30 per cent.

Psychologically a woman may feel that her useful life is over. If children have left home she may suffer from what is commonly called the 'empty nest syndrome', whereby she feels that she is no longer needed.

In fact when viewed from a positive angle it can be seen that the menopause marks a new and interesting phase in life. There is freedom from a number of past responsibilities. Demands on finances may be considerably less. There is freedom from the risk of pregnancy. Quite often there is more time for partners to enjoy each other's company.

## Hormone replacement therapy

It is possible to obtain relief from many of the symptoms associated with the menopause through hormone replacement therapy. It is not a panacea for every woman, nor is it the fountain of eternal youth as some would have you believe. However medical research has found that it has a number of advantages. In geriatric women it is increasingly recognized that hormone replacement therapy can preserve muscle tone associated with the bladder, therefore helping to prevent incontinence. The risk of heart attacks and strokes appears to be reduced.

Progesterones are added to oestrogen for two main reasons:

1  To prevent endometrial hyperplasia and its progression to carcinoma. Progesterones oppose the mitotic or proliferate effects of oestrogen which may lead to endometrial hyperplasia.
2  In sequential therapy to promote a regular and predictable bleed. Progesterones induce secretory transformation, a process which

activates enzymes involved in oestrodial metabolism and endometrial shedding when progesterones are withdrawn. This ensures that menstruation occurs which will bring about the removal of potentially neoplastic cells.

Progesterone may be used in HRT in three ways:

1 As a cyclical monthly course in combination with oestrogen to produce a monthly bleed and protect the endometrium.
2 Continuously with oestrogen – so protecting the endometrium without a monthly bleed.
3 Progesterone only in women who are contra-indicated to oestrogen due to a history of conditions such as breast or endometrial cancer.

There are a number of side effects of oestrogen, namely breast tenderness, nipple sensitivity, nausea, leg cramps, and epigastric discomfort. A few women gain weight.

These side effects can be alleviated with the use of combined oestrogen and progesterone preparations. This is a relatively new concept in the UK but has been used in its various forms for over ten years in North America and Europe.

Dr Robert Greenblatt, an eminent endocrinologist in the United States, believes that the administration of testosterone along with oestrogen enhances the benefit of hormone replacement therapy and frequently eliminates depression. Energy levels and sex drive are improved. There is relief from migraine-type headaches and also considerable improvement in any arthritic condition. Dr Greenblatt also belives that the use of progesterone not only guards against hyperplasia but also against painful breasts, weight gain, and irregular bleeding which may occur when using oestrogen only (*No Change*, Wendy Cooper, 1990).

In a lecture given to members of the Institute of Electrolysis in June 1990 Dr John Studd, Consultant Gynaecologist at King's College Hospital, London, spoke on the use of oestrogen and testosterone in the fight against osteoporosis. There is growing evidence that the use of hormone replacement therapy in the combined form can actively encourage the laying down of new bone. Osteoporosis and its associated complications cost the National Health Service many thousands of pounds each year. It is possible that this cost could be reduced considerably by the use of HRT.

There are a number of other benefits to be obtained from the use of hormone replacement therapy. These include improved muscle tone, firm breasts, supple joints, prevention of dry, wrinkled skin, also healthy hair and nails. Oestrogen helps to maintain the suppleness and elasticity of the vagina, so eliminating painful intercourse.

The main differences between the contraceptive pill and hormone replacement therapy are that the pill uses artificial hormones, whereas hormone replacement therapy mainly uses natural hormones. The contraceptive pill increases hormone levels, whereas hormone replacement therapy replaces the decreased hormone levels.

Hormone replacement therapy does not claim to prevent the aging process or provide instant rejuvenation. What it does do is to slow the whole procedure down, thereby allowing a woman to grow older gracefully and gently.

Therapy may be given in five ways:

1   orally, in the form of pills;
2   transdermal patches;
3   implants;
4   vaginal creams;
5   pessaries.

*Orally*

Hormone replacement therapy may be prescribed for oral use in the form of Premarin, which is oestrogen only, or as a combination of oestrogen and progestogen in the form of Cycloprogynova and Prempak-C. The use of progestogen over a period of 10 to 12 days ensures that any build-up of the endometrium is shed on a regular basis in the same manner as the natural cycle. Oestrogen only is most commonly used for those women who no longer have a uterus. Oral hormone replacement therapy can be varied to meet the needs of the individual.

A dose of oral oestrogens needs to be substantially higher than a non-oral dose. This is because oral oestrogen travels via the portal vein to the liver. A certain percentage is lost in the digestive tract.

*Transdermal patches*

Transdermal patches are small transparent patches impregnated with either:

● Oestrogen only or;
● Combined cyclical HRT, that is, oestrogen and progestogen.

Transdermal patches deliver a constant amount of hormones through the skin. They are usually worn on the lower abdomen, the buttock or the thigh. These patches are replaced at regular intervals (as prescribed by medical practitioner). The advantage of patches is that the hormones are absorbed directly into the bloodstream, thereby avoiding loss in the digestive tract. The disadvantages are that the patch can be easily dislodged and skin irritation may occur. Women who have not had a hysterectomy must use the combined oestrogen and progestogen patches.

Skin reactions at the patch site occurs in up to 30 per cent of women. These can be minimized by applying the patch to the buttock which is less prone to skin irritation, also patches can be applied in a different position every 24–48 hours. Patches which contain alcohol should be left to stand for 10–15 seconds with the backing strip removed before application to the skin. Hot, humid climates increase the possibility of skin reaction.

*Implants*

The hormone implant is a painless, minor surgical procedure. The lower abdomen is anaesthetized. A small incision is made and a metal tube inserted. The appropriate hormone pellets are implanted into the abdominal fat through the tube, then the tube is removed and the incision stitched. The effect of the pellets lasts for up to six months. Some practitioners favour the use of testosterone pellets in addition to oestrogen pellets. It is felt that testosterone may well enhance the benefits of oestrogen. The use of testosterone may cause increased hair growth.

*Vaginal creams*

A number of topical oestrogen preparations are available for short-term relief of dryness and atrophy of the vagina in women who lack systemic symptoms of oestrogen deficiency or who do not wish to go onto systemic treatment.

**Review questions**

1 Name the different phases in a woman's life when major hormonal changes occur.
2 Describe the changes which take place at puberty.
3 Give a detailed description of the menstrual cycle.
4 What is meant by the term 'premenstrual tension'?
5 Explain the benefits that may be obtained from hormone replacement therapy.
6 Name the different ways in which hormone replacement therapy can be administered.

# 8 Gender reassignment

A transsexual is a person who feels very strongly that he/she is trapped in the wrong biological body. The individual is firmly convinced that his/her psychogenic gender is the opposite of his/her anatomical gender. These feelings usually occur at an early stage in life, often before the age of five years. This is not a desire but a desperate need to live and function as the opposite sex.

Transsexuals should not be confused with transvestites. 'Transvestite' is the term applied to men who cross-dress in women's clothes, *from time to time for sexual arousal,* but with no desire to live and function as women. Neither should a transsexual be referred to as homosexual; there are fundamental differences between the two. *Homosexuals enjoy their own sex and prefer to relate to their own gender sexually.* A homosexual man has no desire to undergo surgery, or to live as a woman.

Once experienced, transsexual feelings grow stronger as time goes by. Individuals find it difficult or impossible to suppress these feelings, either through their own efforts or by medical intervention which may include psychoanalysis, psychotherapy, electric shock or the administration of drugs.

There are two constructive courses of action open to these people:

1 to try to adjust to living as best (s)he can as his/her biological sex;
2 to seek gender reassignment (sex change) by surgery.

The decision to go through surgery is not an easy one. There are many emotional, social and physical readjustments to be made, which take place over a considerable period of time. Several barriers have to be overcome before surgery takes place, and a number of adjustments in life have to be made afterwards. The true transsexual must be able to pass successfully as a member of the opposite sex.

## Male to female gender reassignment

There are a number of conditions which must be met before surgery can take place. The person concerned must:

1 undergo considerable stringent psychiatric assessment to establish that they are a genuine *gender dysphoric* (transsexual);
2 be single;
3 be able to live continuously and be self-supporting in their chosen role for a specified period of time, approximately two years;
4 be able to form social relationships as a woman with both sexes;
5 be emotionally stable.

## Male to female surgery

Gender reassignment of male to female involves several hours of surgery. It is a long, slow procedure which can cause many problems unless carried out by a skilful surgeon.

*Surgery involves:*

1   the removal of the testes;
2   the building of a pseudo-vagina;
3   breast enlargement;
4   reduction of the Adam's apple when necessary.

The process is painful and post-operative convalescence may take up to six to eight weeks. It is interesting to note that although the operation is available through the National Health Service in Britain, it is not legally possible to alter the sex stated on the birth certificate, and national insurance records cannot be altered, therefore surgery will have no effect on national insurance contributions or future rights to benefits and pensions. Should a male to female transsexual receive a prison sentence, this will have to be served in a male prison.

Surgery for gender reassignment is available either privately or through the National Health Service. However surgery for breast augmentation, nose reduction and reduction of the Adam's apple are considered to be cosmetic surgery and are not available through the National Health Service.

# Hormone treatment

For two years prior to surgery a programme of hormone treatment will be prescribed. This involves taking oestrogen orally, and possibly an androgen suppressant. Premarin is the usual form of oestrogen prescribed, but in a much larger dosage level than that for the contraceptive pill or hormone replacement therapy. The dosage is usually reduced after surgery.

## *Physiological effects during hormone therapy*

A number of physiological changes take place when hormone therapy is taken over a prolonged period of time. These include:

1   development of small breasts, with pigmentation and enlargement of the areola;
2   increase in, and redistribution of fat cells which affect the contours of the body;
3   improved condition of scalp hair;
4   improvement in skin tone;
5   softening of beard, and hair growth may occur;
6   decrease in size of the testes may occur;
7   long-term impotence and sterility may occur.

*Oestrogen will not:*

1   cause the masculine voice to become more feminine – this can only be helped by speech therapy;
2   decrease or alter beard and body-hair growth;
3   reverse a receding hairline or cure baldness.

# Electro-epilation

The presence of a beard poses many problems for the male to female transsexual who is living and working as a woman. Psychologically it is better to have successfully removed the beard before the operation takes place. To have to continue shaving after surgery has been completed is demoralizing and often leads to severe depression. Adjusting to a new body image after surgery causes enough difficulties without the constant reminder of the pre-operative life.

The only way to successfully eliminate the beard is by electro-epilation. This will be a long, slow process influenced by the density and strength of hair growth, sensitivity of the skin and pain threshold of the individual. The minimum length of time for treatment will be at least two to three years for a light to medium beard growth, and longer for a stronger growth. Duration of treatment will need to be at least two hours a week. Treatment is rarely available on the National Health Service, but for the persistent individual it is sometimes possible.

**Electro-epilation plan for the transsexual client**

It must be remembered that treatment for these clients will be a long slow procedure. As previously mentioned it is better to start treatment as soon as possible before surgery, in order to clear as much hair growth as possible prior to gender reassignment.

Length of treatment can expect to take 18 months to two years before surgery, and up to a further three years after surgery. Two hours a week is advisable, with the time decreasing as progress is made.

**Treatment procedure**

1  Starting at the ears gradually work downwards on sideburns and sides of face to thin the hair out.
2  Work downwards on cheeks. At this stage it is better to ignore regrowth, and concentrate on fining down the texture in order to tone down the blue shadow.
3  Proceed to the chin and upper lip. Care must be taken to avoid over-treatment of the upper lip. By this stage the electrolysist should be able to gauge the skin's response to treatment and work accordingly.

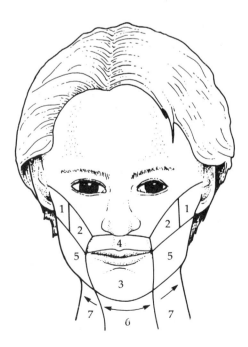

**Figure 8.1** Treatment procedure

4  Progress to the neck and jaw line, gradually moving down to the sternum and breast area.

It will still be necessary for the transsexual client to shave between treatments. Psychologically, the sooner the hair growth can be diminished the better. It must be remembered that these clients will be living and working in their female roles for some considerable time before surgery takes place. The presence of a beard is both embarrassing and socially unacceptable.

At least two hours a week should be allowed for treatment, with one hour concentrating on hair that has not been treated and one hour devoted to regrowth.

With *careful planning and conscientious work* the skin will not be harmed. Method of treatment depends on the individual's skin reaction. The author has found the Blend method to be the most effective treatment for these clients. Due to the nature of the hair growth the use of more galvanic than normal may be necessary, i.e. up to 1 mA, and therefore the use of cataphoresis at the end of the session is advisable in order to neutralize the surface effect of sodium hydroxide. When treating with shortwave diathermy there is a risk of pigmentation due to the high levels of oestrogen being prescribed.

The importance of the correct home and after-care routine must be stressed. Advice on skin-care routine and products to improve the condition of the skin is often necessary.

The electrolysist will probably become more of a confidante than with any other client, and can help with tips on make-up and leg waxing etc. When the transsexual client is living and working in her new role the electrolysist is often the only person with whom she can discuss her problems and difficulties.

It can be seen from the preceding text that gender reassignment is not an easy option. The procedure involves a complete change of life style, which may mean loss of family and friends; also a change of career or job may be necessary. The decision requires courage and a great deal of determination.

**Review questions**

1  Explain the difference between a transsexual, transvestite and homosexual.
2  What are the conditions which must be met before surgery for male to female reassignment can take place?
3  Describe the hormone treatment which is necessary prior to surgery.
4  State the physiological effects which occur during hormone therapy.
5  Give a treatment plan for the transsexual client.
6  Explain the complications that may arise due to the amount of treatment required by a transsexual client.

# 9 Needles

The correct choice of needle plays an important role in the successful destruction of the lower follicle and dermal papilla. The function of the needle is twofold: firstly it acts as a probe, allowing the needle to slide smoothly and easily into the follicle, secondly it acts as an electrode, allowing the current to flow evenly to the tip of the needle. A good quality needle should have a smooth, polished surface with a well-defined, yet rounded tip.

How often do operators give a thought to the development and quality of the needle they are using, or the effect the needle has on the efficiency of the treatment not to mention the comfort of the client? The history of the epilation needle is fascinating and much of the early information that is available to electrologists to date can be attributed to the meticulous and thorough research undertaken by Derek Copperthwaite, Editor of *International Hair Route Magazine*, Canada.

It is recorded that when Dr Charles Michel conducted his first experiments into hair removal using galvanic current he used a fine no.8 sewing needle. The original needles used by Dr Michel were in all probability produced by one of the many needle factories to be found in and around the Redditch area of England.

The demand for epilation needles in the early days was very small. The American distributors of medical equipment looked towards fine sewing needles which were being imported from Europe. At that time the demand for electrolysis needles was insufficient to justify the expense involved in producing a specialized tool. It was found that a fine sewing needle could be adapted by either leaving out the eye or cutting it off altogether. Needle holders were made from wood or hard rubber.

In the late 1880s Daniel Mahler (founder of the still thriving Instantron Company, Rhode Island), was using fine English darning needles similar to those used by Dr Michel. Some fifty years were to pass before there was sufficient demand to warrant the manufacture of a specialized needle.

Initially these needles were produced from sewing needles, manufactured in Redditch, England. The diameter was approximately .010 of an inch, the length being in the region of 2.5 inches. Needles were buffed and polished by hand, usually four at a time, on a jewellery polishing wheel. A somewhat tedious task. Needles were not produced from stainless steel and therefore had to be coated with Vaseline to prevent them from staining and rusting.

One of England's first companies to specialize in the manufacture of quality needles was founded by a man called MacKenzie, in Whitechapel, London. MacKenzie's needles soon gained a reputation for being the finest, strongest and best in the trade. Unfortunately MacKenzie got into severe financial difficulties and was forced out of business by his creditors. Around this time Alcester in Warwickshire became the better known home of needle production, and trade in London declined.

The following description is reproduced from the *International Hair Route Magazine* by kind permission of author and editor, Derek Copperthwaite:

Accurate Records from 1852 describe the manufacture of needles as follows:

A coil of steel wire is cut into lengths sufficient to make two needles: these lengths are collected into bundles, and straightened by a special process. The grinder then takes a number of the pieces in his hand, and points them (at each end on a dry grindstone). They are now washed, and dried over a fire.

The next process is done by children: about 50 of the wire lengths are fastened down to a strip of wood and then passed to a workman at another machine - powered by a treadle under the man's foot – where a file is moved over the needles to remove any imperfections.

From here the needles go to a kind of vice, and the upper part of the double-ended needles are worked backwards and forwards until they break in two at the middle. The tops of the heads are now filed round, and any roughness removed.

The needles are then hardened by placing them in a furnace until they are red hot. From there they are emptied into a tub containing oil or water and then tempered by being placed over a slow fire and allowed to cool gradually. Any crooked needles are straightened with a small hammer, one at a time, on an anvil.

Mixed with oil, soft soap, and emery powder, the needles are then wrapped in a sackcloth and placed in a kind of mangle, worked by mill power, to be scoured. This process takes about a week, and when done the needles are washed in hot water and dried in saw dust. Winnowing and sorting follow. The points are then set and the needles polished on a leather buffing wheel.

At the time this description was written, upwards of 10,000 people in England were employed in the needle manufacturing industry. Altogether, in its making, each simple needle passed through the hands of 70 or more workmen and under-went ten or more separate operations. In 200 years of needle making since then, the factories of Redditch have produced billions of needles.

Today's needles are produced in factories using automated equipment and thankfully the procedure is considerably less labour intensive.

Prior to 1981, when the first pre-sterilized needles were launched, electrologists main concerns were the durability of the needles; how long they would last and what was the most effective way to sterilize needles for re-use. The autoclave that we use today was not available.

The most common practise was to turn the electrolysis machine up to full intensity. A piece of cotton wool was first soaked with surgical spirit and then held with a pair of tweezers. The needle was then inserted into the cotton wool between the tweezers and a sharp burst of high frequency current was applied to it. Needless to say with the advent of AIDS and hepatitis this method is no longer acceptable. The arrival of the sterile disposable needle has proved to be a valuable asset to electrologists in the UK and many other countries. Many local authorities within the UK insist on the use of disposable needles before granting a licence to practise.

The way electrologists work today was changed in 1981 when Sterex International launched the first pre-sterilized epilation needle. This was shortly followed by pre-sterilized needles from Arand Ltd with Ballet needles and the Carlton Professional needle of Taylor Reeson Laboratories.

Features of pre-sterilized needles include:

- Medical grade packaging.
- Sterilization by gamma irradiation or eythel oxyene gas.
- Needles are packed individually either in single pouches or tear off strips.

The main reason for the interest in disposable needles was the possible risk of cross infection from AIDS and hepatitis. Manual sterilization of needles is time-consuming, and there is a risk of inadequate sterilization if the procedure is not carried out thoroughly. Up to February 1990 there have been three documented cases of acupuncture-related AIDS.

The first sterile disposable needle was introduced by Sterex in 1981, the needles initially being imported into England from the USA. These needles were then packaged individually and sterilized by gamma irradiation. Due to the increase in demand, Doug Cartmell and John Heath commenced the manufacture of Sterex needles in England. These are now exported widely. Needle diameters range from 003 to 006, with the addition of 010 for the treatment of warts and skin tags.

During 1988 the 'Ballet' needle was launched by Joseph Asch of Arand Ltd. Before entering the electrolysis market Arand had specialized in the exportation of high-quality sterile needles for use in medical surgery and acupuncture. Many prototypes were designed before Arand Ltd were finally satisfied with the quality.

The Ballet needle is constructed of a single piece of highly-polished stainless steel, packed in hospital grade blister packs and sterilized with ethylene-oxide gas. For sensitive skins this needle is also available in 24 carat gold plate, bonded evenly on to the needle surface. The needle diameter is available in 002, 003, 004, 005, 006. The 002 needle is very fine, proving particularly useful for facial and upper lip work or where the client is worried by fine vellus hair.

In February 1989 Carlton Professional entered the market with a two-piece flexible needle, diamond drawn from austentic stainless steel and finished with a final polishing process. Each needle is fitted with a protective plastic cap, individually packed and sterilized by gamma irradiation. Needle diameters are 003, 004, 005, 006. This needle took 19 months to develop as opposed to the six months originally envisaged.

For electrical epilation a good quality needle should have a smooth polished surface (see Figure 9.1) which will facilitate insertion into the follicle. When the surface is smooth the current will flow evenly to the tip of the needle. This is due to the fact that the current will flow to the point of least resistance. Where the surface is rough the current dissipates at the roughened surface, therefore less concentration of current reaches the tip of the needle where it is required (see Figure 9.2). Current intensity will have to be increased in order to destroy the papilla and lower follicle effectively. This results in a more painful treatment for the client.

The next consideration is the shape of the needle point/tip. Tests have shown that with a micro-polished rounded point, current intensity can be lowered significantly (see Figure 9.3). Should the needle point be rough,

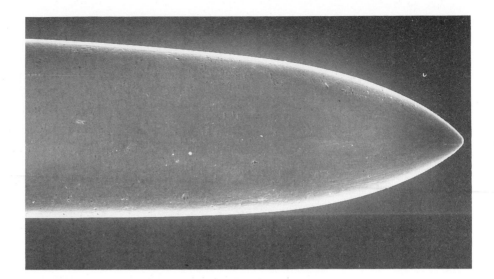

**Figure 9.1** Smooth
needle surface

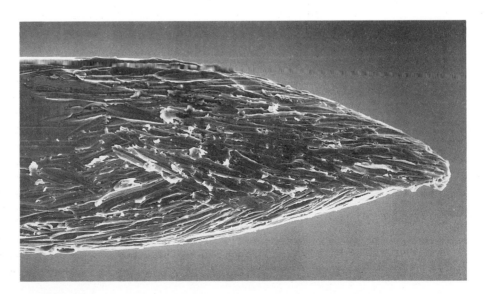

**Figure 9.2** Rough
needle surface

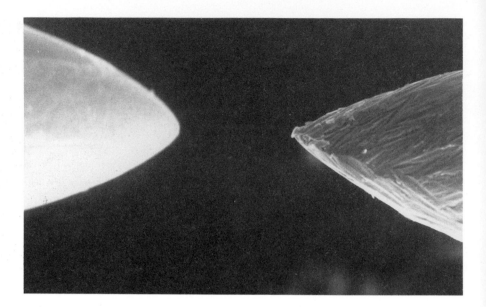

**Figure 9.3** *(left)* Rounded point; *(right)* Sharp point

micro-lesions to the follicle can result, which hinders the healing of the skin after treatment.

When the point of the needle is blunt easy entry into the follicle is hindered (see Figure 9.4), whereas when the point is too sharp the risk of piercing the follicle wall, or probing through the base is increased.

Further considerations when choosing the needle are, the diameter, length and shape. The diameter of the needle should match the diameter of the hair, i.e. the coarser the hair, the larger the needle – this enables the tip of the needle to encompass the base of the follicle, so enabling the current to reach the entire area requiring treatment. Should the diameter of the needle be too small, the intensity during high-frequency application is concentrated in a small area, which is more painful to the client. There is also a risk of under-treating the follicle, due to insufficient current reaching the entire base. When the diameter is too large the follicle wall could be stretched and result in broken capillaries.

Needles can be obtained in both regular and short lengths. Should the needle be too short it may not be possible to reach the base of deeper follicles, so resulting in insufficient electrical action to the target area.

There are five types of needle available:

1 one-piece tapered needle;
2 two-piece – straight;
3 two-piece – tapered;
4 insulated;
5 24 carat gold plated.

## One-piece tapered needle

This needle is constructed from one piece of stainless steel which is highly polished to give a smooth surface (see Figure 9.5). There is less risk of the needle breaking or separating from the shank. When the needle is tapered,

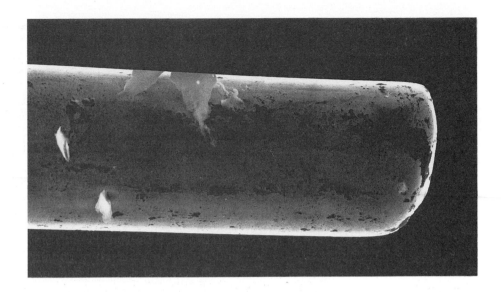

**Figure 9.4** Blunt
needle

the current, be it galvanic or high frequency, is concentrated at the narrowest point, which will be the tip of the needle. In other words there will be low current density at the larger area and higher current density at the tip – where the action is needed – therefore the risk of over-treating upper follicle and epidermis is reduced

These needles are available in two shank sizes – F and K. The K shank is more widely used in European countries and partly in America and Australia. The F shank fits most British, American and Australian needle holders.

## Two-piece needle

The two-piece needle is constructed from stainless steel, using a fine piece of steel running through a stainless steel shank (see Figure 9.6). This construction allows more flexibility. The two-piece needle is available in both straight and tapered shapes. Availability varies in different countries.

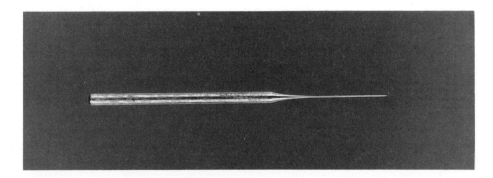

**Figure 9.5** One-piece
needle

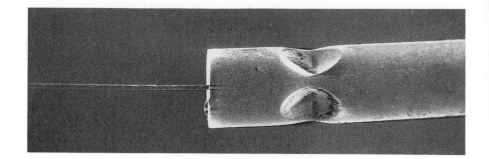

**Figure 9.6** Two-piece needle

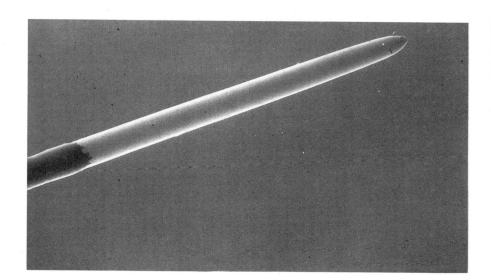

**Figure 9.7** Insulated needle

## The insulated needle

The insulated needle consists of a needle coated with an insulating material which leaves ⅟₂₅ inch (1.0 mm) of the needle exposed (see Figure 9.7). Traditionally, the disadvantage of insulated needles is that the insulation makes the needle thicker, and the insulation is inclined to lift away from the needle after sterilization, so hindering insertion. There may also be a slight risk of deposits of insulation in the hair follicle.

In the spring of 1991 Ballet introduced the first disposable insulated needle. The insulating material is a modern polymer that is only 0.00004 in (one micron) thick. This minimal addition makes a totally imperceptible difference to the electrolysist.

The advantage of insulated needles is that the current is concentrated at the tip of the needle, and is therefore ideal for sensitive skin. Because the needle is only used once, and the polymer is extremely smooth and hard, the insulation remains on the needle.

***Gold plated needles***

The gold plated needle consists of a stainless steel tapered needle, which has had 24 carat gold plate bonded on to the entire needle surface. The addition of cobalt gives gold a little bit of strength. Gold is an excellent conductor of electricity and does not oxidise with age. It is a slippery metal, which aids ease of insertion.

This needle is ideal for people who are sensitive to stainless steel. Swelling and erythema are reduced, both important benefits in all electrical epilation treatments, including the treatment of telangiectasia.

# Review questions

1 Name the two methods used for sterilizing disposable needles.
2 State the advantages of using disposable needles.
3 What are the requirements of a needle when used for electrical epilation?
4 What effect does a rough needle surface have on current distribution?
5 Why should the diameter of the needle match the diameter of the hair?
6 State the purpose of an insulated needle.
7 What are the advantages of a gold plated needle for sensitive skins?

# 10 Electricity

Electricity has a number of uses. It may be used to produce heat, cold by refrigeration, light, or chemical changes by various processes, e.g. galvanic electrolysis. Without electricity electro-epilation cannot take place.

The wise electrolysist will be familiar with the basic principles and applications of electricity for a number of reasons.

1  Safety and efficiency may be increased, with less risk of damaging equipment, giving or receiving an electric shock, or overloading the system.
2  By understanding the effects of applying galvanic current and high frequency to the hair follicle and skin, the operator is able to decide which method of electro-epilation will be most suitable for the area and type of hair to be treated.
3  By understanding the process taking place in the follicle and skin during current application, it is possible to avoid damage to clients through over-treating, or incorrect application.
4  Additional benefits may be the ability to carry out minor repairs such as changing fuses, repairing cables to needle holders, changing plugs, etc. The need to call in an electrician for routine maintenance or minor repairs may be eliminated, as may costly bills and loss of income through equipment being out of commission. It should be stressed however that unless the electrolysist is indeed skilled in these areas a suitably qualified technician or electrician *must* be called in.

## What is electricity and how can it be used to advantage in the salon?

Electricity is often referred to as either static or dynamic. It is static electricity which builds up on our hair after vigorous brushing, so causing the hair to crackle and fly away; it is also static electricity which results in a mild shock from an object such as a light switch or car door in which a build-up of excess electrons has occurred. This form of electricity is said to be 'at rest'.

Dynamic electricity is a controlled flow of energy formed from the movement of electrons. It is electricity in motion, e.g. direct and alternating currents.

A simple definition by explanation of the electrical terms commonly used with most equipment in galvanic treatment is given below:

An *electrolyte* is an alkaline or acidic solution, which allows the conduction of an electric current. Moisture in the skin, which is mildly acidic, enables the current to pass from the needle into the skin tissue. Tissue fluids in the body are electrolytes.

An *electrode* is the conductor, which is used to make contact with the electrolyte. During electro-epilation the needle acts as the electrode and allows the current to flow into the moisture within the hair follicle and skin tissue. When using a direct current, two electrodes are necessary to form a complete circuit.

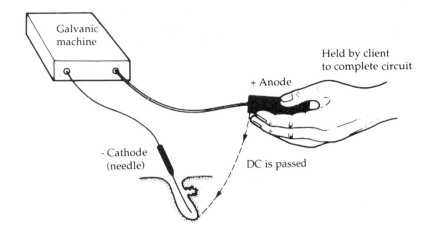

+ Anode

Held by client
to complete circuit

Galvanic
machine

- Cathode
(needle)

DC is passed

**Figure 10.1** Direct current from machine to client

*Polarity:* a direct current possesses polarity because it flows in one direction only, through a complete circuit. To achieve this the current requires two poles, one negative and the other positive, in order to form a circuit. The electrically charged electrons which form the current flow from negative to positive (see Figure 10.1).

*Ionization* occurs when a direct current is passed through an electrode into an electrolyte. During electrolysis the salt molecules contained within the body tissues separate into electrically-charged ions. The electrolyte solution will allow the movement of positively-charged cations towards the cathode (negative electrode), and the movement of negatively charged ions towards the anode (positive electrode).

The *anode* is the positively charged electrode. During electrolysis the anode is held by the client. It is known as the indifferent electrode. The anode is connected to the positive outlet of the galvanic machine.

*Cataphoresis* occurs when the active anode repels positively charged cations into the skin. This procedure may be carried out using either a roller, rod or tweezer electrode. It is usually applied at the end of an epilation treatment by galvanic electrolysis.

The *cathode* is the negatively charged electrode, which becomes active during electrolysis. The cathode is connected to the negative outlet of the galvanic machine.

*Anaphoresis* is the result of the active cathode repelling negatively charged anions into the skin. As with cataphoresis, a roller, rod or tweezer would be used, usually at the beginning of an epilation treatment.

*Electrolysis* this term, when used in connection with permanent hair removal, refers to a chemical process which takes place when a direct current is applied to tissue salts and moisture contained within the hair follicle and surrounding skin tissue. As a result sodium hydroxide is produced which destroys the tissue because it is highly caustic.

Having followed the current from the machine, through the needle holder and probe into the follicle, consideration should be given to the process which takes place. This makes it necessary for the electrolysist to understand about atoms and molecules etc. These may be defined as follows:

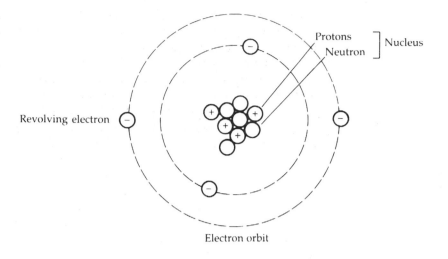

Proton = positive charge
Electron = negative charge
  An atom contains an equal number of protons and electrons
    An atom is neither positively nor negatively charged

**Figure 10.2** The atom

**a** Sodium chloride (salt) molecule

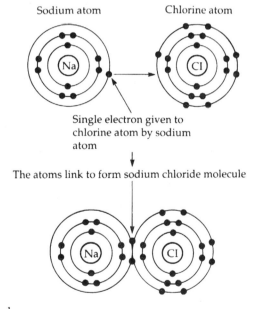

**b** Water molecule

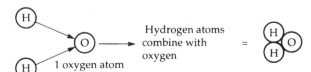

**Figure 10.3** The
formation of a molecule

*Atoms* an atom consists of a central nucleus containing neutrons and positively charged protons. Neutrons are electrically neutral. Usually the number of neutrons equals the number of protons. The overall number of neutrons does not affect the electrical charge of the atom. Negatively-charged electrons rotate around the protons. When the number of electrons and protons are equal the atom is neutral (see Figure 10.2).

*Molecules* are the smallest units into which a substance can be broken down without losing its basic properties. It is possible to divide molecules into atoms. The properties of the individual atoms may be very different to those of the molecule they form, e.g. two atoms of hydrogen and one atom of oxygen combine to become one molecule of water. The properties of water are entirely different from those of hydrogen and oxygen in their separate entities (see Figure 10.3).

*Ions* are formed as a result of an atom either losing or gaining an electron. A positively-charged cation is formed when an atom loses an electron, whereas a negatively charged anion is formed when an electron is gained.

The basic principle of attraction and repulsion can be used to explain the exchange of electrons:

Electrons – negative
Protons – positive

Opposites attract, whereas like repels. Therefore an electron will be attracted to a proton, whereas two electrons will move away from each other (see Figure 10.4).

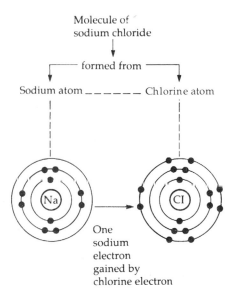

Molecule of
sodium chloride

⎯ formed from ⎯

Sodium atom _ _ _ _ _ _ Chlorine atom

One
sodium
electron
gained by
chlorine electron

Sodium atom has lost an electron thereby having one more proton than electrons. The electrical charge is therefore POSITIVE and becomes a sodium Ion-Na⁺

Chlorine atom has gained an electron thereby having one more electron than protons. The electrical charge is therefore NEGATIVE and becomes a chloride Ion-CI⁻

**Figure 10.4** The formation of ions

## Electric currents used in electro-epilation

*Direct current* (dc) is a flow of electrons along a conductor in an electric circuit of constant voltage. A direct current possesses polarity. The current flows in one direction and destroys hair by chemical reaction within the tissues.

*Alternating current* (ac) reverses its direction of flow at regular intervals, thereby changing polarity within the circuit (unlike direct current which flows in one direction only). A *cycle* refers to one complete alteration, or change of direction, the *frequency* means the number of complete cycles per second, and *Hertz* is the term used for a complete cycle (see Figure 10.5).

*High frequency* is used in electro-epilation to destroy tissue by the heat it produces. It is a high-frequency, low-voltage, alternating current, ranging from 3–30 million cycles per second, or 3–30 MHz. Theoretically a higher frequency, lower voltage should produce a more comfortable treatment for the client. In practice much depends on the sophistication of the circuit design.

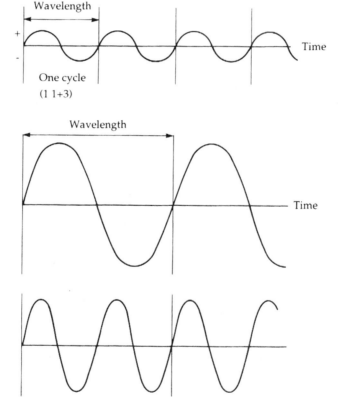

**Figure 10.5** Alternating currents

## Components used in electro-epilation equipment

The most central part of equipment is the power supply. This is used to convert electricity from the domestic supply into that of the right voltage and type, i.e. ac or dc, for the rest of the electronic or electrical equipment within the appliance (see Figure 10.6).

**Figure 10.6** Components used in electro-epilation equipment

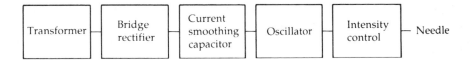

| Transformer | Bridge rectifier | Current smoothing capacitor | Oscillator | Intensity control | Needle |

The basic components used in a simplified power supply are shown above. More modern designs will usually have more sophisticated forms of voltage regulation and may use a technique called a switch mode regulation. However, for the purpose of understanding most equipment and the basic components this example will be adequate.

The *transformer* changes the voltage of an alternating current. It can either step-up/increase the voltage, or step-down/decrease the voltage, and is generally used to convert the domestic supply voltage to that required by the equipment.

The *rectifier* is a device consisting of two or more diodes which changes an alternating current to a direct current. A diode allows the current to flow through it in one direction only. The bridge rectifier, containing four diodes, is more efficient.

The *capacitor,* which may also be known as the filter or condenser, is used to smooth out the bumps in a direct current which has been produced by a rectifier.

The *voltage regulator* prevents the voltage surging, or suddenly increasing, if the client's resistance becomes lower during treatment.

The *rheostat* (variable resistor) also known as the variable current control regulates the output of current from the machine to the needle (usually by controlling the voltage regulator circuit).

The *constant current generator* maintains the current at the pre-set level despite any change in resistance (of the client being treated).

# Conductors and non-conductors

A *conductor* is a substance such as steel, copper or, in the case of electro-epilation needles, stainless steel or gold, which allows an electric current to flow when electric pressure is present in a given direction. Other examples of conductors are zinc, carbon and impure water (see Figure 10.7).

A *non-conductor* prevents the current from passing *along* it; examples are wood, plastic, rubber and glass. A non-conductor can also be referred to as an insulator.

The *cable* of the needle holder demonstrates the use of both a conductor – which is the copper wire contained in the centre – and a non-conductor, or *insulator*, which is the plastic coating surrounding the wire.

**Figure 10.7** Flex and needle holder indicating a conductor (copper wire) and insulator (covering material)

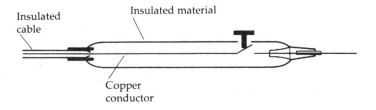

Insulated cable

Insulated material

Copper conductor

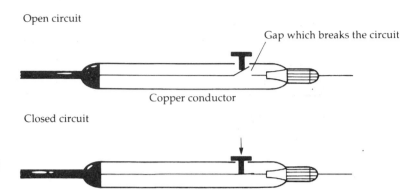

Open circuit

Gap which breaks the circuit

Copper conductor

Closed circuit

**Figure 10.8** Open and closed circuits

## Circuits/circuit breakers and fuses

### Circuit

A circuit can be defined as the path taken by an electric current. The circuit may be closed to allow the current to flow, or open to prevent it flowing.

Fuses, switches and other overload devices may intentionally be used to open the circuit and prevent the current flowing in the event of a malfunction such as a short or equipment failure, thereby protecting both the client and the operator (see Figure 10.8).

An open circuit exists when the flow of current has been interrupted, usually by a switch, but sometimes as a result of broken wires contained within the flex.

### Circuit breaker

This is a switch which breaks the flow of current when the circuit becomes overloaded. Its function is to prevent damage to the circuit or equipment through an overload of current. The switch is activated by thermal contact. When the intensity of current is too high the circuit is broken. The circuit breaker serves the same function as the fuse, the difference being that the switch can be reset whereas the fuse must be replaced.

### Fuses

The fuse is designed to be the weakest link in an electrical circuit. When too high an intensity of current is passed the fuse will blow (melt) thereby breaking the circuit and preventing further current flow. The purpose of a fuse is to act as a safety device to prevent an overload of current to a piece of equipment, or possible damage to another part of the wiring. A faster-acting and safer method of protection is the earth leakage contact breaker.

The *cartridge fuse* is used in all flat-pin plugs. It consists of a porcelain or glass tube containing the fuse wire soldered to a metal contact cap at each end. The fuse is held in position by metal clips connected to the live terminal. When the fuse is blown the complete cartridge is replaced. The correct fuse value should be used at all times. The most widely used fuse values/ratings are 3 amp, 5 amp and 13 amp.

The *mains fuse:* The older-type mains fuse box contains porcelain fuse holders. A piece of fuse wire is connected by a screw at each end of the holder. The fuse rating will depend on the type of circuit it is protecting, e.g. lighting, power sockets or electric cooker. When this type of fuse blows only the wire is replaced. It is always advisable to keep a card of fuse wire and a screwdriver next to the mains fuse box. Later boxes have thermal/magnetic circuit breakers and cartridge fuses, which may be manually reset.

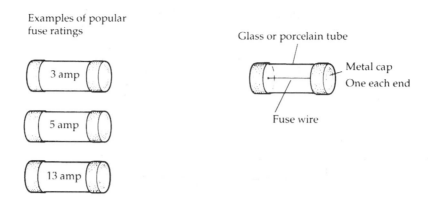

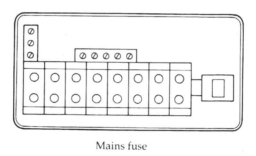

**Figure 10.9** Cartridge fuses

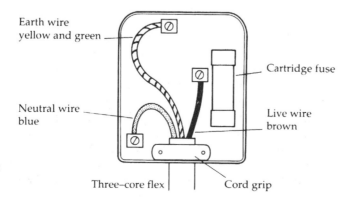

Mains fuse

# Wiring of a three-pin flat plug

The neutral wire is blue and should be connected to the left-hand side of the plug.

The live wire is brown and is always connected to the terminal next to the cartridge fuse.

The earth wire is green and yellow. It is connected to the terminal at the top of the plug. The purpose of this wire is to act as a safety device, taking any excess or stray electricity to earth, so preventing any person who is using the equipment from receiving a shock. Not all appliances contain a three-core flex. Some are designed with 'double insulation', allowing them to function safely with a two-core flex which will contain a blue and brown wire for connection to the neutral and live terminals. *Where an earth wire is provided, it must be connected on a three-wire flex.*

Earth wire yellow and green

Cartridge fuse

Neutral wire blue

Live wire brown

**Figure 10.10** Wiring of a three-pin flat plug

Three–core flex

Cord grip

The cord grip on a plug is designed to hold the outer casing of the flex firmly and help prevent the wires from working loose.

The wiring in a plug should be checked regularly to ensure that the wires are all still firmly connected to the relevant terminals.

## Units of electrical measure

**Ampere**   Measurement of the intensity of current. It is the rate of electron flow and is expressed in coulombs. The strength of the current is equivalent to a flow of one coulomb per second equals one amp.

**Coulomb**   The measurement of an electrical charge.

**Milliampere**   One thousandth of an ampere. It is the unit most frequently referred to in electro-epilation.

**Watt**   A unit of electrical power. One watt of power exists when one ampere is felt at a pressure of one volt.

**Volt**   A measurement of electrical pressure.

**Voltage**   Measures the potential difference between two points of a circuit. The force produced by a battery or generator pushes the electrons, and thereby the current round the circuit.

**Ohm**   The measurement of resistance. Conductors offer less resistance to electrical pressure than non-conductors.

**Ohm's law**   It takes one volt to push a current of one ampere through a conductor with a resistance of one ohm. This may be expressed as $V = IR$.

## Review questions

1   Define the following terms:
   (i) electrolyte
   (ii) electrode
   (iii) polarity
   (iv) ionization.
2   Describe each of the following:
   (i) atom
   (ii) molecule
   (iii) ion.
3   What is the difference between dc and ac?
4   (a) Name the components found in electrical epilation equipment.
   (b) Briefly describe the purpose of each component.
5   Define the following:
   (i) circuit
   (ii) circuit breaker.
6   Compare the cartridge fuse with the mains fuse.
7   Draw and label a diagram to show the wiring of a three-pin plug.
8   What is the purpose of the cord grip in a plug?
9   Define the following units of electrical measure:
   (i) ampere
   (ii) milliampere
   (iii) volt
   (iv) voltage.
10   Define Ohm's law.

# 11 Galvanic electrolysis

The permanent removal of unwanted hair by means of electrical epilation owes its reputation to the thoroughness of galvanic electrolysis.

The history of electrolysis can be traced back to 1875 when Dr Charles Michel of St Louis, Missouri, reported to medical colleagues that after applying a negatively charged galvanic current to the follicle the hair did not regrow. In time it was realized that the follicle had been permanently destroyed by the action of sodium hydroxide.

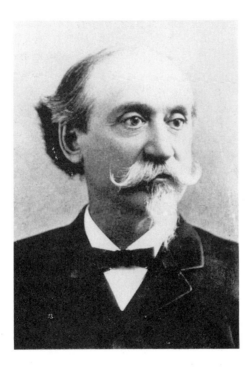

**Figure 11.1** Dr Charles Michel

Skin specialist Dr Hardaway followed this discovery in 1876 by using electrolysis for non-medical purposes. The year 1880 saw the publication of *Electricity in Facial Blemishes* – the author Plymouth S. Hayes, MD. Hayes indicated that it was possible to guarantee the permanent removal of hair by means of galvanic electrolysis.

During 1886 a further publication entitled *The Use of Electricity in the Removal of Superfluous Hair* was written by Dr George Henry Fox. Dr Fox was one of the more sympathetic medical practitioners of that time where superfluous hair was concerned. He was aware that although excessive hair growth did not kill the patient it certainly had a detrimental effect on her mental health and well-being.

However galvanic electrolysis had a number of drawbacks. Application time of current to the follicle took from between one to three minutes to

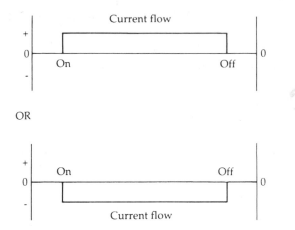

**Figure 11.2** Direct current

Constant current flow in one direction only with no change in polarity

remove the hair. This made the treatment slow, tedious and impractical for an extensive hair growth.

The machines used in these early days were not as refined as those used today. The direct current was produced by batteries, the intensity was often higher, and was therefore more painful for the client. A greater degree of skill was needed to operate these machines correctly in order to avoid skin damage or an excessively strong current being passed.

An extensive build-up of sodium hydroxide occurred in the tissues due to the length of time the current needed to flow. The result was widespread tissue destruction, and in many instances scarring.

In 1916 Professor Kree developed the multiple needle technique. This method speeded up the process by using up to 10 needles at any one time. The needles used then were much larger, with the surface being rougher.

Due to the many drawbacks, galvanic electrolysis was gradually replaced by shortwave diathermy.

## The galvanic current

The galvanic current, discovered by Luigi Galvani, is a *direct current* (see Figure 11.2). It is a flow of electrons along a conductor in an electric circuit. When a direct current passes through an electrolyte which contains ions, the ions move in opposite directions. The ions carry the current.

Electrolysis can be defined as a chemical process which occurs when a direct current is applied to:

1 tissue salts and moisture; or
2 salt-water solution.

The direct current causes the salts and water to split into their chemical elements, which then rearrange themselves to form entirely new substances. During the passage of direct current through salt-water solution the negative chloride ions (anions) are attracted to the positive anode, and the positive sodium ions (cations) are attracted to the negative cathode. When the chloride ions reach the anode they lose an extra electron to become chlorine atoms. Sodium ions arriving at the cathode gain an

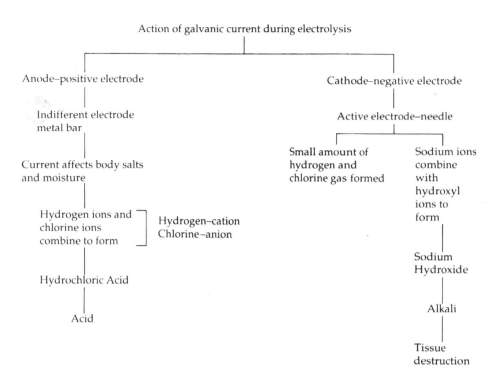

**Figure 11.3** Action of galvanic current during electrolysis

electron and become sodium atoms. The sodium atoms react with water to form sodium hydroxide, while the chloride ions form hydrochloric acid.

The electrodes used during electrolysis are known as the anode, which is positive, and the cathode, which is negative. Negatively-charged anions are attracted to the positive anode, whereas positively-charged cations are attracted to the negative cathode. The principle is that like poles repel one another and unlike (or opposite) poles attract each other.

## How does galvanic electrolysis take place?

During the application of galvanic current to the lower follicle chemical changes take place (see Figure 11.3). Moisture and body salts are composed of molecules. These molecules are formed of atoms which divide under the influence of galvanic current. The ions regroup and are converted into sodium hydroxide, hydrogen gas and chlorine gas. This process takes time to develop in the follicle. Sodium hydroxide is not produced immediately but is dependent on the intensity of the current used, together with the length of time the current flows. Therefore:

current intensity × length of application = amount of sodium hydroxide

One tenth of a milliamp of current flowing for one second will produce one unit of sodium hydroxide. Therefore the longer the time and/or the greater the current intensity, the more sodium hydroxide will be produced. The electrolysist needs to bear this principle in mind when selecting the current intensity and time for application. Full details are given in Chapter 13.

All hairs of a similar type may be treated with one setting. Obviously, more sodium hydroxide is needed for coarse, deep, terminal hairs and less

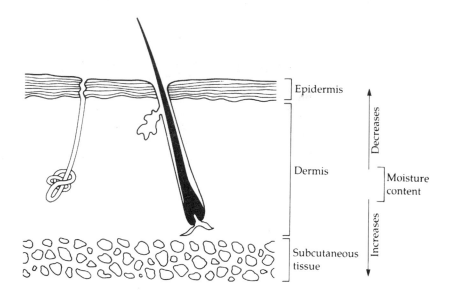

**Figure 11.4** Moisture gradient of the skin

for fine, medium or shallow hairs. Size of hair, moisture content of skin, and stage of hair growth all have an effect on the treatment.

## Effect of electrolysis on the hair follicle

When using galvanic electrolysis, destruction of the hair and follicle is achieved in the following way: The indifferent electrode is attached to the positive outlet and handed to the client. This may be covered in damp viscose or damp lint.

The needle holder is connected to the negative outlet.

A small amount of negatively charged current is applied to the lower follicle through the needle. When the current encounters moisture within the tissues a chemical action takes place and sodium hydroxide is formed. This chemical action is not instantaneous, but takes time to develop. It does not stop the moment the needle is removed from the follicle, but continues to work for a short time afterwards. The amount of sodium hydroxide produced depends on three factors:

1   the length of time the current is flowing;
2   the intensity of the current used;
3   the moisture content of the skin.

The direct current is available along the entire length of the needle but it affects tissue *only* where moisture is present.

## Moisture gradient

As previously mentioned, the presence of moisture is necessary before electrolysis can take place. The skin has the advantage of encouraging electrolysis action to take place at the base of the follicle, where it is required, due to its natural moisture gradient. The concentration of moisture in the skin is higher in the deeper layers of the dermis, gradually decreasing nearer to the epidermis (see Figure 11.4).

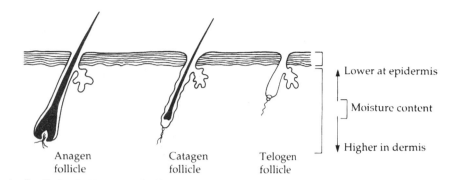

**Figure 11.5** Follicles

| Anagen follicle | Catagen follicle | Telogen follicle |

Lower at epidermis

Moisture content

Higher in dermis

### *Moisture in relation to follicle depth*

The hair growth cycle also has a part to play in successful application of galvanic electrolysis. During anagen the follicle grows down into the deeper layers of the dermis – here the concentration of moisture is good. As the follicle progresses to catagen, the follicle begins to collapse and retreat upwards thereby moving away from the higher concentration of moisture. In telogen, the active parts of the lower follicle have completely collapsed, leaving only the dermal cord (see Figure 11.5). The resting follicle lies close to the skin's surface, where the moisture content is very low or absent.

Vellus hair lies close to the skin's surface. Treatment of this type of hair is more successful with shortwave diathermy rather than blend or galvanic electrolysis, for two reasons:

1  the lack of moisture;
2  the presence of sebum.

*Sebum* is an excellent insulator. Therefore the sebum present in the upper follicle protects the epidermis from galvanic action taking place close to the skin's surface (see Figure 11.6).

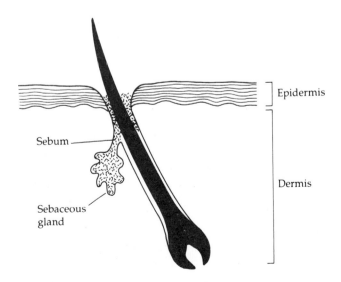

Epidermis

Sebum

Dermis

Sebaceous gland

**Figure 11.6** Sebum-insulating property

| Needle<br>Negative (-) | Needle<br>Positive (+) |
|---|---|
| **Action** ||
| Cathode | Anode |
| Negative charge | Positive charge |
| Sodium hydroxide | Hydrochloric acid |
| Tissue destruction without discolouration | Tissue destruction |
| | Disintegrates steel needles black oxide deposits |
| | Tissue discolouration black tattoo marks in skin |
| Any scar tissue formed will be supple | Any scar tissue formed will be hard |

**Figure 11.7** Effect of current application to follicle using a needle

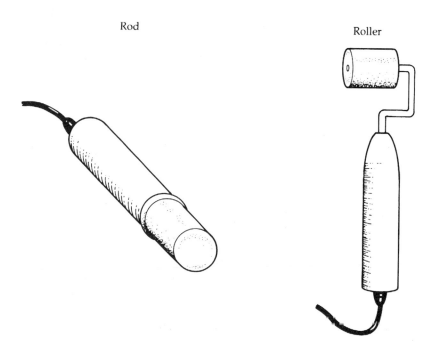

Rod

Roller

**Figure 11.8** Current application to skin surface using rollers or rod

Moisture content and moisture gradient of the skin vary from one person to another and from one area of the body to another. It can be affected by exposure to winds and sunlight, harsh cosmetic preparations, illness or certain medications.

# Effects of polarity

The effects of the polarity on the skin will differ depending on how the current is applied.

## Current application to follicle using a needle

When using a needle as the active electrode the current is concentrated in a very small area and will result in tissue destruction. It is essential that the needle is only ever used with the *negative* electrode (see Figure 11.7).

## Current application to skin surface using rollers

When the current is applied to the skin's surface using a roller or rod (see Figure 11.8) the effects will be less concentrated and give a different result. The cathode (negative roller) will:

1  soften and relax skin tissues;
2  irritate nerve endings;
3  produce erythema due to vasodilation;
4  produce skin ionization, causing irritation.

This process, referred to as anaphoresis, can be usefully employed before electrolysis when the follicles are tight. Due to the relaxing of skin tissues the follicles open slightly, making insertion easier.

When the anode (positive roller) is used, the opposite effects are achieved:

1  skin tissue is firmed;
2  the superficial blood vessels are constricted, reducing erythema in the area;
3  nerve endings are soothed, which is pleasant for the client and induces a feeling of well-being;
4  hydrochloric acid is formed, which neutralizes the effect of sodium hydroxide and helps to restore the skin's pH balance;
5  skin de-ionization occurs.

Cataphoresis (using anode) is beneficial after treatment or when a client's skin is sensitive to galvanic treatment.

# Electrolysis equipment

Batteries are no longer used in electrolysis. Today's machines operate from the mains. The main components in the machine are:

1  transformer;
2  rectifier;
3  capacitor;
4  regulator (voltage);
5  variable current control;
6  a number of machines contain a meter which indicates the milliamp reading.

Coming from the machine will be:

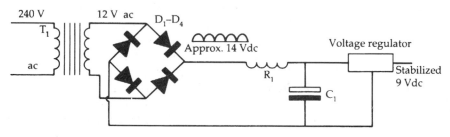

T$_1$ = Transformer
D$_1$–D$_4$ = Rectifying diodes
R$_1$ = Current limiting resistor
C$_1$ = Current smoothing capacitor

**Figure 11.9** Alternating current (ac) to direct current (dc)

Voltage regulator or equivalent electronic circuit set to adjust final voltage to that required

1   negative outlet;
2   positive outlet;
3   current intensity (milliamp) control.

An alternating current of 240 volts enters the machine and is then changed into a smooth direct current of up to 100 volts. Most if not all electrolysis machines use no more than 30 to 40 volts dc. This change takes place in the manner described below (see Figure 11.9).

1   The alternating current is passed through a transformer which reduces, or steps down, the voltage. The transformer also acts as a mains isolation.
2   The current is then changed from alternating current to direct current by the bridge rectifier.
3   The (filter) capacitor smooths out any irregularities in the direct current.
4   The filtered/smoothed current goes through a voltage regulator. The constant voltage generator is built in, to ensure that the voltage stays stable while the current intensity (ma) is varied in accordance with the required setting. The purpose of this is to prevent the current surging or suddenly increasing in intensity should the client's resistance to the current become lower during treatment.
5   The variable current control regulates the current output from the machine to the needle.

**Treatment procedure**

1   Sanitize the area to be treated.
2   Hand the positive stainless steel electrode to the client, who should be asked to maintain a firm hold to prevent fluctuation of current flow during treatment. The electrode may be covered in wet cotton wool or sponge. This will help the conduction of the current.
3   Insert pre-sterilized needle into the needle holder.
4   Probe follicle.

5  Apply current, gradually increasing intensity to client's tolerance level. This will normally be between 0.2 and 0.5 milliamps depending on the type of hair growth to be treated.
6  Check the length of time taken to loosen the hair. This will probably be between 30 and 90 seconds, but may be considerably longer.
7  Remove treated hair from follicle.
8  Continue treating hairs of similar type.
9  At the conclusion of the treatment apply aftercare.

When the treatment has been completed cataphoresis may be applied to the area. For this procedure the negative electrode is handed to the client. The positive electrode, which may be a stainless steel or carbon roller, is moved gently over the skin for several minutes.

The effect of cataphoresis is to reduce erythema; the hydrochloric acid produced neutralizes the effects of sodium hydroxide; nerve endings are soothed, thereby promoting a sense of well-being and relaxation in the client.

## *Progressive electrolysis*

Progressive electrolysis is the method by which operators work with both hands simultaneously (see Figures 13.15-13.17). The right-handed operator holds the electrolysis probe in the right hand, the tweezers are held in the left hand. The needle is inserted into the follicle. The galvanic current is activated, the hair is then held with the tweezers (without tension) and the current allowed to flow until the hair releases. The hair is lifted gently every few seconds and if the hair is not ready to release the tension is relaxed. When sufficient lye has been produced the hair will slide easily out of the follicle. Time, practise and patience is required to master this technique.

## Review questions

1  Define 'galvanic current'.
2  Define the term 'electrolysis'.
3  Describe what happens when a direct current is passed through a saline solution.
4  Define the following:
   (a) anode; (b) cathode; (c) cation; (d) anion.
5  Describe how sodium hydroxide is formed in the follicle.
6  What is the effect of sodium hydroxide on the follicle?
7  How does galvanic electrolysis take place?
8  Name three factors which affect the production of sodium hydroxide in the hair follicle during galvanic electrolysis.
9  What is meant by the term 'moisture gradient'?
10  How is electrolysis affected by the moisture gradient in relation to the skin?
11  In what way does sebum affect the application of galvanic current?
12  Compare the effects of galvanic current applied through the needle on:
   (a) the negative charge; (b) the positive charge.
13  List the effects of: (a) anaphoresis; (b) cataphoresis in galvanic electrolysis.

14  What are the benefits of applying cataphoresis to the skin after galvanic electrolysis treatment?

15  List the disadvantages of galvanic electrolysis.

16  Describe the treatment procedure for galvanic electrolysis.

17  State the main advantage of galvanic electrolysis.

# 12 High-frequency treatment

**History**

The use of high frequency for electrical epilation came into being because galvanic electrolysis was slow, painful and resulted in a high percentage of scarring.

Many people making valuable contributions over the years were responsible for the development of high frequency and its eventual use in electrical epilation. The principal pioneers included the following:

*Heinrich Hertz* was the first scientist to demonstrate the existence of high frequency. Hertzian waves were named in his honour.

*Professor Arsene d'Arsonoval of Paris* discovered that it was possible to introduce Hertzian waves into the body at oscillation frequencies of 100,000 cycles per second without causing muscle stimulation.

*Guglielmo Marconi* discovered radio waves in 1896 through the radiation of electrical energy into space.

*Van Zeyneck* observed in 1899 that organic tissue could be heated by high frequency.

*Dr Bordier of Paris* wrote the first article on the use of high frequency for the removal of hair.

During the 1940s shortwave diathermy treatment, using high-frequency, superceded galvanic electrolysis. Initially it appeared to be a much faster and more effective method. However the main disadvantage is the higher percentage of regrowth.

**High frequency voltage**

High frequency is an oscillating alternating current of very high frequency and low voltage. This ranges from 3–30 MHz or 3–30 million cycles per second.

The high-frequency value describes the number of times the current completes a cycle each second. Every frequency has a fixed wavelength. As the frequency increases the wavelength decreases. Thus the wavelength of a 13.56 MHz wave is twice that of a 27.11.062 MHz (see Figure 12.1).

Due to the possibility of radio waves generated by electrical epilation units interfering with radio and television transmissions, countries have

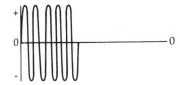

**Figure 12.1**
Frequencies

allocated and standardized specific permitted frequencies. Many countries use 13.56 MHz. CTI's Blendette 48-ACM uses 40.68 MHz.

## Epilation equipment

The following terms are often referred to in electrical epilation:

1 shortwave diathermy;
2 radio frequency or RF;
3 thermolysis and high frequency, or HF;

The explanation for these terms is straightforward. Epilation equipment utilizes the short-waveband radio frequencies. When applied to the follicle, thermolysis occurs, that is, tissue is destroyed by the heating effect caused by the agitation of molecules in the surrounding tissue.

An epilation machine consists of the following components (see Figure 12.2):

1 an oscillator which may be formed from a capacitor and inductor, and/or crystal;
2 a power supply to drive the oscillator;
3 a variable intensity control.

Crystal oscillators are used in a number of instances, stabilizing the capacitor/inductance design. The advantage of this type of oscillator is that each crystal oscillates at its natural frequency regardless of environmental conditions, whereas capacitor/inductance type oscillators can be affected by several factors such as humidity, temperature, material and component quality. What this means is that capacitor/inductance oscillators can have a wide fluctuation in frequency. The tolerance of the inductance/capacitor oscillator also determines the tolerance of the frequency. In contrast, crystal oscillators can have an accuracy in excess of 0.001 per cent.

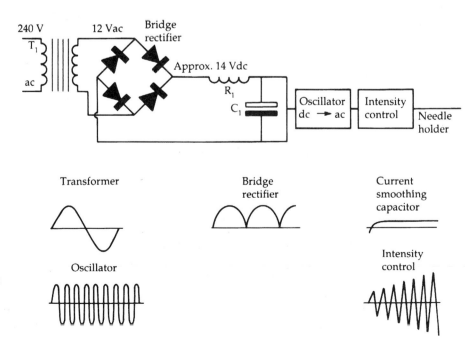

**Figure 12.2** Progress of current in high-frequency epilation machine

In a capacitor/inductance type oscillator a 'variable or tuning' capacitor is used to vary the coupling of the oscillator to the needle holder output socket in order to control the output intensity of the machine. In a crystal control oscillator the same is achieved by varying the amplitude of the oscillator signal.

Inductance/capacitor type oscillators have a maximum frequency of 18 MHz. In crystal oscillators where the higher frequency is selected by the manufacturer, for example in excess of 27.12 MHz, factors including the length of the cable to the needle holder, and cable impedance, are critical. These factors affect the efficiency of transfer of energy from the generator to the needle tip.

## Production of heat by high frequency

During the application of high frequency to the follicle the electrovalency of molecules within the tissues is altered. The rapid agitation of atoms causes the atoms to vibrate against each other which results in friction. This in turn causes a temporary release of energy in the form of heat. It is the moisture within the tissues which is heated — not the needle.

The heating pattern commences at the sharpest point of the needle (which should be the tip) where the high-frequency energy is most intense, gradually building up around the needle. The term 'high-frequency field' is used to describe the heating pattern radiating from an epilation needle, connected by a wire to a high-frequency oscillator. The 'high-frequency field' is strongest close to the needle, and in practice will concentrate around the needle tip.

## Effect of heat on tissue

Heat destroys tissue either by cauterization or by coagulation.

Cauterization occurs when a high intensity of high frequency is passed into the tissue. The moisture vaporizes and the tissue becomes dry. Coagulation occurs when a lower intensity of high frequency is used. The cellular structure in the tissue breaks down and protein is congealed. Electrical epilation should aim at coagulation of the lower hair follicle, to bring about destruction without damaging the surrounding tissue.

## Heating pattern

The heating pattern is the shape of the heated area surrounding the needle during the application of high frequency. The heating pattern will develop only where moisture is present. The ideal development of heat is pear shaped, commencing at the tip of the needle and gradually building up around it (see Figure 12.3).

A number of factors influence the successful application of high frequency in the follicle:

1　needle diameter;
2　quality of needle surface;
3　needle depth;
4　application time of high frequency;
5　intensity of high frequency;
6　moisture content and gradient;
7　correct and accurate insertion.

### Needle diameter

The needle diameter should equal the diameter of the hair to enable the tip of the needle to encompass the base of the follicle. Should the needle be

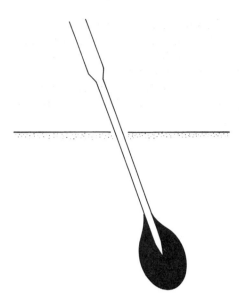

**Figure 12.3** High-frequency heating pattern

too small, the intensity will be concentrated on a smaller area. This is often more painful to the client (due to the concentration of high frequency to a smaller area) but does not give sufficient high frequency to the area being treated. If the diameter is too thick, the follicle wall could be stretched, thereby bruising the skin and possibly causing broken capillaries (see Chapter 9).

*Needle depth*

Should the insertion be shallow, the high frequency will be applied too close to the skin's surface. This could result in surface burns and blistering. With shallow insertions, the high frequency misses the base of the follicle and therefore permanent destruction will not occur. Should the insertion be too deep the base of the follicle will be penetrated and the high frequency will be applied to tissues below, which will result in the destruction of deeper tissue, eventually leading to pit marks and scars. (See Figure 12.4.)

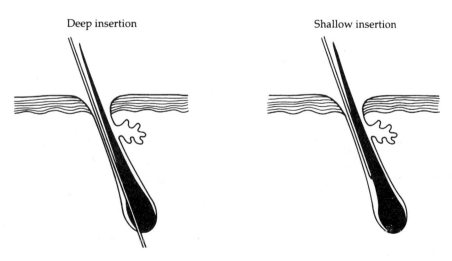

Deep insertion          Shallow insertion

**Figure 12.4** Needle depth

**Application time of high frequency**

The effect of time on the heating pattern should be considered. The heating pattern starts at the tip of the needle, progresses up the shaft and at the same time expands in width around the tip where the concentration of high frequency will be highest. If the high frequency is applied for too short a time, insufficient heat will be generated. Should application be too long, the heating pattern will eventually reach the skin's surface, resulting in scars. (See Figure 12.5.)

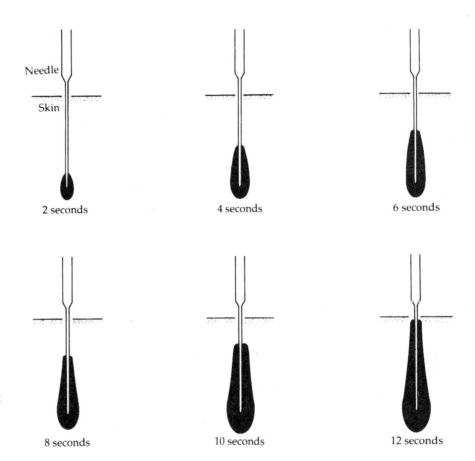

Needle

Skin

2 seconds

4 seconds

6 seconds

**Figure 12.5** The effect of time on high-frequency heating pattern

8 seconds

10 seconds

12 seconds

**High-frequency intensity**

When intensity is too low, tissue coagulation will take longer, therefore application time will need to be increased. When the current intensity is higher, the heating pattern will commence at the tip of the needle, gradually building upwards. The aim is to use the highest intensity setting that the client can comfortably tolerate, yet at the same time bring about tissue destruction by coagulation, not by cauterization.

**Moisture content of skin**

As with galvanic electrolysis, the moisture gradient has an effect on the application of high frequency to the follicle. The concentration of moisture is higher in the deeper layers of the skin, so helping to limit the action of the high frequency to the lower half of the follicle. Problems can occur when the client's skin contains a high surface moisture content. Skill by the operator is required in order to keep the electrical action at the base of the follicle. With a skin which has a high moisture content it is possible that the high-frequency action could reach the surface before sufficient destruction has taken place in the lower follicle.

## Treatment procedure

1  Sanitize area to be treated.
2  Insert sterile disposable needle into needle holder.
3  Turn on machine!
4  Probe follicle.
5  Apply sufficient high frequency to remove hair easily without causing an adverse skin reaction. The current intensity should be set within the client's pain threshold.
6  Remove treated hair with sterile tweezers. The hair should slide out of the follicle without traction.
7  Continue treating hairs of similar type, adjusting high-frequency intensity when necessary.
8  At the conclusion of the treatment apply suitable aftercare.

## Flash technique

Flash refers to the application of a very high intensity of high frequency to the follicle for a fraction of a second. Due to the short duration of high frequency application the client's nerve endings do not have time to respond, therefore less pain is experienced. The two methods of high-frequency application differ in tissue destruction and heating pattern.

With flash technique the heating pattern is narrow, rising up the follicle quickly (see Figure 12.6), whereas a lower high frequency setting produces a pear-shaped heating pattern expanding from the needle tip. Tissue destruction by flash is brought about by desiccation, in other words the heat produced dries out the moisture and burns tissue, whereas a lower high-frequency intensity applied for a longer period of time breaks down cellular protein and results in tissue destruction by coagulation.

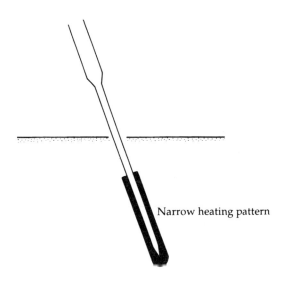

Narrow heating pattern

**Figure 12.6** Flash technique

**Review questions**

1   Define 'high frequency'.
2   Explain the meaning of the following terms associated with electro-epilation:
    (a) shortwave diathermy;
    (b) radio frequency;
    (c) thermolysis.
3   (a) Name the main components used in a shortwave diathermy machine.
    (b) Describe the function of each of these components.
4   Explain how the high frequency current creates heat within the follicle.
5   What is the effect of heat on the skin tissues?
6   Explain how tissue destruction is achieved by:
    (a) coagulation;
    (b) cauterization.
7   Draw a diagram to illustrate the ideal heating pattern when high frequency is applied to the follicle.
8   List the factors which influence the successful application of high frequency in the follicle.
9   List the disadvantages of using the incorrect needle size during electro-epilation.
10  How does the quality of the needle surface affect the efficiency of electro-epilation treatment?
11  Describe the effects on the skin when the needle depth during treatment is:
    (a) too shallow;
    (b) too deep.
12  How does intensity affect application time of the high frequency.
13  How does the skin's moisture content affect application of electro-epilation?
14  What is meant by the 'flash technique'?
15  What are the disadvantages of using flash technique?

# 13 Blend

The blend technique is an exciting development which enables the electrolysist to treat superfluous hair more effectively. The high percentage of regrowth experienced with shortwave diathermy is reduced, the length of time taken to clear an area is reduced, and subsequent scarring, which often results when using galvanic alone, is eliminated.

The blend came into being due to the foresight and efforts of Henrie St Pierre and Arthur Hinkle. Pioneer electrolysist Henrie St Pierre was dissatisfied with the length of time taken to destroy hair permanently with galvanic, or the high percentage of regrowth experienced with high frequency. He joined forces with Arthur Hinkle (author of *Electrolysis, Thermolysis and the Blend*) who at this time was an electronics engineer. Both felt that there must be a way of combining both methods in order to achieve the advantages of each technique.

**Figure 13.1** (left)
Henrie St Pierre

**Figure 13.2** (right)
Arthur Hinkle

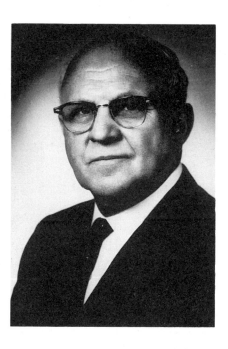 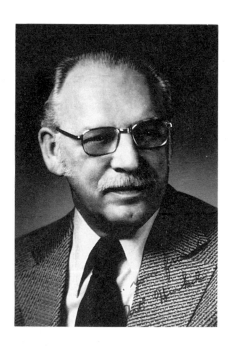

Work on the blend technique commenced in 1938. A patent was applied for in 1945 and granted in 1948. The technique has now been established for many years in countries such as the USA, Canada, Holland and New Zealand.

Blend was introduced into Britain in the early 1980s by Norman Harris with the Thermagal machine. Joan Thornycroft, well known and respected for her work on the education boards of CIBTAC and CIDESCO invited specialists in the field from Holland to run the first comprehensive Blend

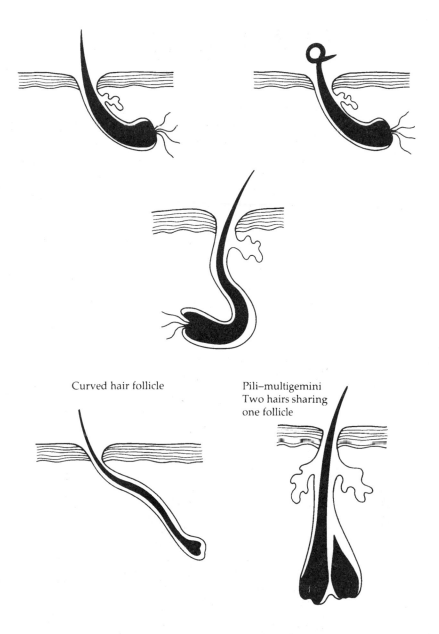

Curved hair follicle

Pili–multigemini
Two hairs sharing
one follicle

**Figure 13.3** Examples of distorted follicles

course in Britain during 1980. However it was not until 1988 that general interest began to take hold and British companies began the development of blend machines for the UK market.

The principle of the blend is to enhance the chemical action of galvanic electrolysis with the simultaneous application of high frequency.

## How does blend work?

The application of the two currents works in the following way: both currents are present at the needle, either separately or together, with each retaining its own characteristics and identity. The dual or blended action takes place within the follicle. The galvanic current brings about tissue destruction by chemical action, whereas high frequency produces heat to speed up the chemical action brought about by the galvanic current. (High frequency when used in shortwave diathermy destroys tissue by heat.)

The blend is a versatile epilation method that can be adapted to treat most hairs effectively including curved or distorted follicles and deep bulbous hairs. Blend requires approximately 75 per cent less time to provide the same degree of destruction as galvanic electrolysis alone. It is faster than galvanic but slower than high frequency.

*Curved or distorted follicles* are unsuitable for treatment by high frequency (see Figure 13.3). Due to the fact that the tip of the needle cannot be placed accurately at the base of the follicle, the high-frequency heating pattern is unable to reach the dermal papilla and base of the lower follicle. The sodium hydroxide produced during blend, being fluid, can move easily into any open space that will accommodate a liquid.

The successful application of the blend technique relies upon the correct balance between the two currents. When used together, galvanic and high frequency currents are superimposed. Both currents are available at the needle either separately or together as required. Each current *retains* its own true form and is not changed by the presence of the other current. The tissue is affected by each current in the following way:

- *Galvanic current:* electrons flow along the needle into the hair follicle. When making contact with tissue and moisture within the follicle a chemical reaction takes place. Sodium hydroxide is produced and, being highly caustic, destroys the surrounding tissue.
- *High frequency current:* the rapid oscillations of the high frequency current cause vibrations of water molecules within the tissue. This results in friction which in turn causes heat. *The action of sodium hydroxide is accelerated by heat.*

The action of the two currents is blended in the tissue. The combination of the action from both the currents is more effective than the 'sum' of the separate actions.

## Action of high frequency during blend application

The action of high frequency current in the follicle enhances that of galvanic electrolysis in three ways.

1 Heat produced by high frequency breaks down the cellular structure of the follicle, causing the protein to congeal. The congealed tissue becomes porous which allows the passage of sodium hydroxide into the tissue.
2 High frequency (oscillation) creates turbulence, so forcing galvanically produced sodium hydroxide into the porous tissue.
3 The heat produced increases the action of sodium hydroxide, thereby shortening the time needed to destroy the lower follicle. Heated sodium hydroxide is two to 16 times more effective in destroying tissue than galvanic electrolysis.

When the balance of the two currents is not correct during treatment the results will not be as good. When too much galvanic current is used the advantages of high-frequency speed are lost – there is less causticity, porosity and turbulence due to the decreased heat produced. Over-treatment of

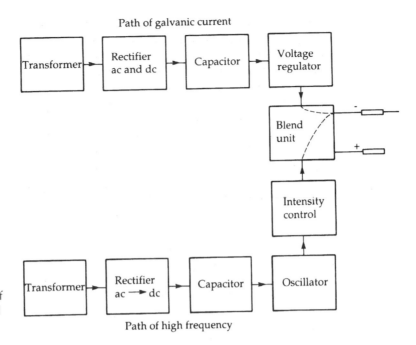

Path of galvanic current

**Figure 13.4** Progress of ac and dc during blend treatment

Path of high frequency

skin will result in weeping follicles. Should too much high frequency be used the effect would be to cauterize the lower follicle, less galvanic action would be produced, and therefore less sodium hydroxide. Over-treating will result in blanched skin.

The combination of the two currents can reduce the application time of galvanic to between six and 15 seconds, the average being 10 to 12 seconds on most machines. With a number of modern machines the time is reduced to between six and eight seconds. A minimum of six seconds is necessary in order to achieve the blended action of both currents in the follicle. Under six seconds does not allow sufficient production of sodium hydroxide.

Much depends on the client's pain tolerance. The treatment appears to be less painful than either current used individually. The combined currents seem to have a numbing effect on the nerve endings.

When applying the current it is advisable to cover the indifferent electrode, which the client holds, with damp cotton wool or sponge. This prevents irritation to the skin due to the build-up of hydrochloric acid which forms at the anode. The thinner the electrode, the more intense the irritation.

## The blend epilator

The blend epilator (see Figure 13.4) consists of the following components: for the galvanic part there will be the transformer, rectifier, capacitor, regulator, milliamp meter, negative outlet, positive outlet and current intensity control. The high frequency will require an oscillator consisting of capacitor and inductor or crystal, plus a current intensity control.

Accessories will be the needle holder and possibly a foot switch, a cable connecting the needle holder to the machine, a metal or carbonized rubber electrode for the client to hold, and a roller for the application of phoresis at the beginning and end of the treatment. Another useful addition is an air pump which when activated injects sterile air through the needle holder

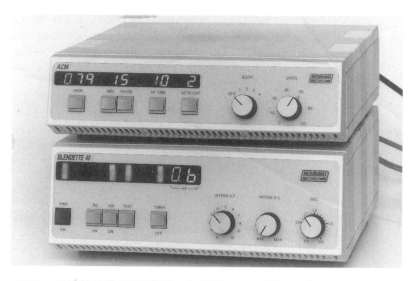

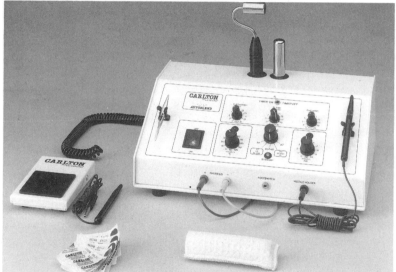

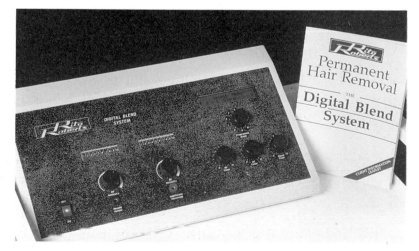

**Figure 13.5** CTI Blendette 48 ACM (top); Carlton Professional (middle); Rita Roberts Digital Blend Unit (bottom)

in coordination with the application of the high-frequency and galvanic currents. This has a mild desensitizing or numbing effect on the skin.

Some machines use two foot pedals to regulate the current, whereas others use one. Others utilize a finger switch control.

Advanced features found in a number of machines include: automated current settings and timings, insertion sensor, moisture level test, desensitizing air, galvanic after-count, hair counter, high-frequency timer which will eliminate inaccurate counting, and body technique facilities.

## Units of lye

To make life easier for the electrolysist Arthur Hinkle introduced the term 'units of lye'. Lye is the popular name given to sodium hydroxide. The amount of lye required to destroy a hair permanently will differ according to the type of hair, depth of follicle, stage of hair growth and area being treated. The stronger, deeper hairs require more lye than shallow, vellus hairs. All hairs of a similar type may be treated identically.

The rate of lye production is directly related to the amount of current being used. Lye is not produced instantaneously but takes time to develop in the follicle. A simple formulation adapting Faraday's law is:

Tenths of a milliamp × time in seconds = units of lye

i.e. five-tenths of a milliamp × 3 seconds = 15 units of lye

Electrolysis produces lye on a very small scale within the follicle. It takes one-tenth of a milliamp flowing for one second to produce one 'unit of lye'. Therefore, the amount of lye produced in the hair follicle is the product of current intensity used, times the length of time the current flows. The longer the time and/or the greater the current intensity, the more lye will be produced. See Table 13.1.

Table 13.1   Guide to units of lye

| | |
|---|---|
| Fine, unpigmented vellus hair | 10–15 units |
| Fine, pigmented, soft hair | 10–20 units |
| Medium/shallow terminal hair | 15–30 units |
| Deep terminal hair | 30–45 units |
| Very deep terminal hair | 45–60 units |

## Determining the balance of the blend

The aim of the blend is to achieve complete destruction of the lower follicle, including the dermal papilla, in the shortest possible time.

It is the high-frequency current which determines the length of time the blend is applied to the follicle. Care must be taken to avoid using the high frequency at too high a setting, which would be to the detriment of the blend technique. The application time is affected by:

1   client's pain tolerance;
2   the sensitivity of the skin;
3   the type of hair growth, e.g. fine, medium, coarse;
4   the stage of follicle development.

The production of lye is affected by the milliamp setting and depth of insertion. A shallow insertion reduces the amount of current flow and therefore the amount of chemical action. With deeper insertions more chemical action will occur due to the higher concentration of moisture in the lower layers of the skin.

## Establishing the current setting for the blend

*Determine the number of seconds required to loosen hair with high frequency.*

Using high frequency only, establish a 'working point' that will give the correct high-frequency setting. This will be a lower setting than used for diathermy.

### Method A

Count the number of seconds needed to loosen the hair. Divide high-frequency settings into units of lye to give galvanic setting in milliamp tenths, e.g. three seconds of high frequency (hf) divided into 15 units of lye (ul) equals five milliamp tenths (ma), or 0.5 milliamps (see Table 13.2).

**Table 13.2**

| Seconds of hf | divided into | Units of lye | Milliamp tenths DC | Milliamps |
|---|---|---|---|---|
| 5 | divided into | 15 | 3/10 | 0.3 |
| 15 | divided into | 30 | 2/10 | 0.2 |
| 6 | divided into | 30 | 5/10 | 0.5 |
| 5 | divided into | 30 | 6/10 | 0.6 |
| 9 | divided into | 45 | 5/10 | 0.5 |
| 5 | divided into | 45 | 9/10 | 0.9 |
| 10 | divided into | 60 | 6/10 | 0.6 |
| 6 | divided into | 60 | 10/10 | 1.0 |

Note: from the client's point of view, with stubborn hairs it is better to increase the length of time during which high frequency is applied rather than to increase the galvanic milliamp setting.

### Method B

*Find dc threshold level.* Insert probe into follicle. Turn on dc, gradually increasing the current. When the client's tolerance level has been reached, stop current flowing and check milliamp reading.

Calculate the length of time needed to treat the hair. Divide units of lye by milliamp tenths, e.g. 0.5 ma on legs requiring 60 units of lye: 60 u/l divided by 5 milliamp tenths = 12 seconds.

## Variations of blend application

1 Having determined the high-frequency intensity, apply both currents simultaneously, then finish with an after-count of galvanic. The purpose of this is to encourage sodium hydroxide to fill the follicle on removal of the hair. This method is the most widely used in Holland, Germany, the United States, Canada and Japan.

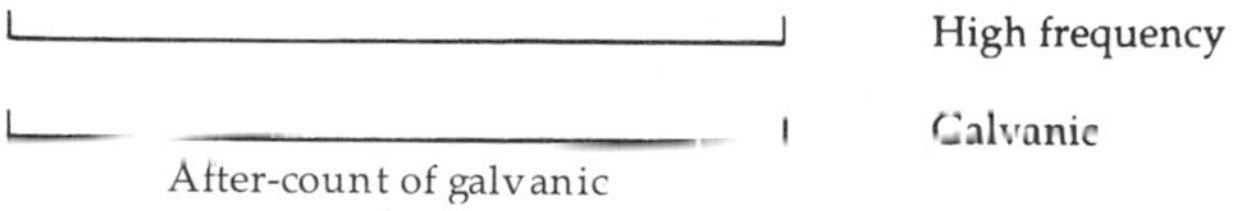

High frequency

Galvanic

**Figure 13.6** After-count of galvanic

After-count of galvanic

2 *Simultaneous application of both currents* during the entire application to the follicle.

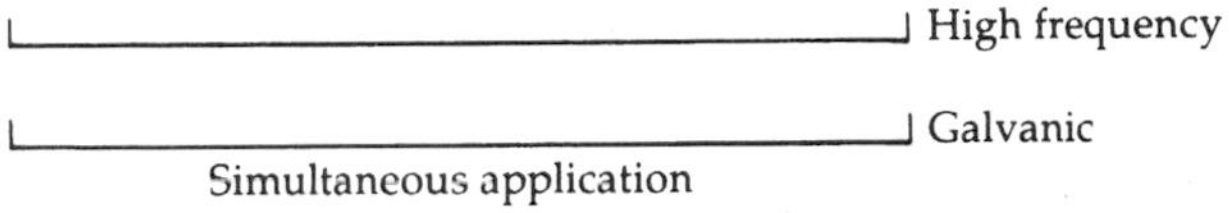

**Figure 13.7** Simultaneous application

High frequency
Galvanic
Simultaneous application

3 *Start with high frequency* then apply both currents simultaneously. The purpose of this is to warm the follicle slightly and also numb the nerve endings. When using this variation it is essential that the high-frequency intensity is not too high, otherwise the moisture in the follicle will be removed and this in turn will prevent the formation of sodium hydroxide.

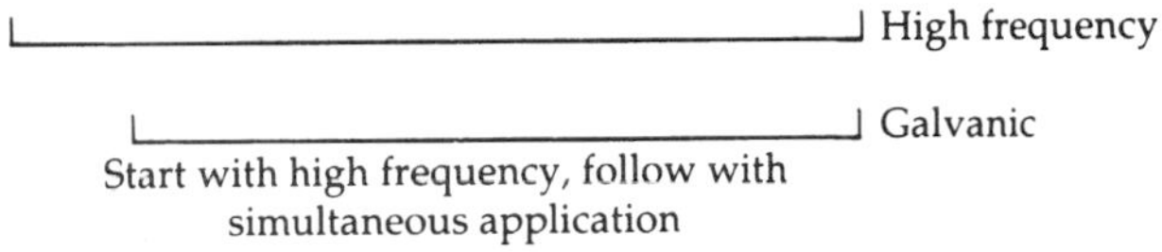

**Figure 13.8** Start with high frequency, follow with simultaneous application

High frequency
Galvanic
Start with high frequency, follow with simultaneous application

4 *Lead with high frequency* to warm the follicle slightly and numb the nerve endings, follow with galvanic current to commence quick production of sodium hydroxide in the pre-warmed environment, then apply both currents simultaneously.

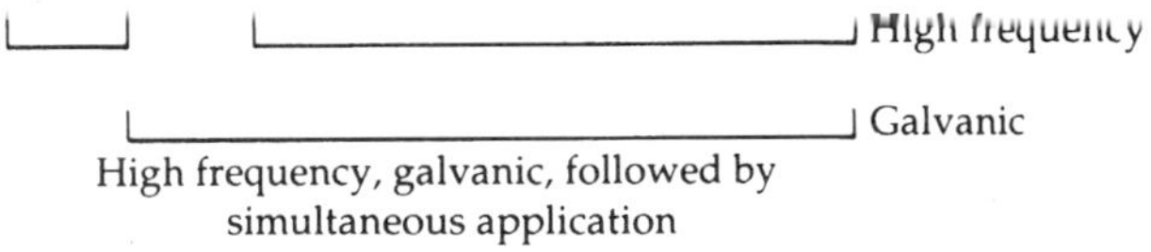

**Figure 13.9** High frequency, galvanic, followed by simultaneous application

High frequency
Galvanic
High frequency, galvanic, followed by simultaneous application

5 *Start with galvanic current* to commence production of sodium hydroxide, then follow with both currents.

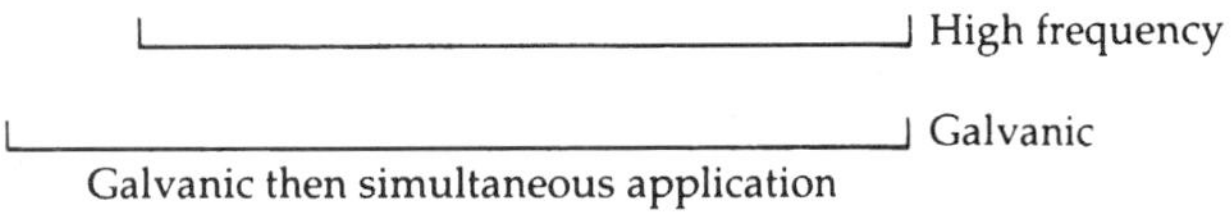

**Figure 13.10** Galvanic then simultaneous application

High frequency
Galvanic
Galvanic then simultaneous application

6 *Lead and finish application with galvanic*, apply both currents together in the middle of current application. This last method is a combination of (1) and (5).

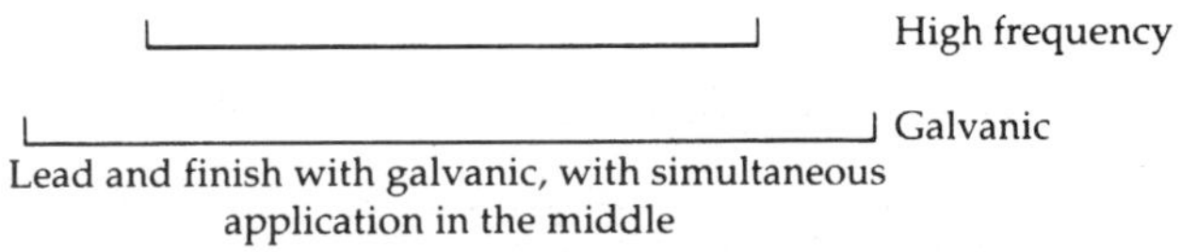

**Figure 13.11** Lead and finish with galvanic, with simultaneous application in the middle

High frequency
Galvanic
Lead and finish with galvanic, with simultaneous application in the middle

## Treatment procedure

1 Remove any make-up or lipstick in the immediate area. Prepare and sanitize area to be treated.
2 Give the sponge-covered positive electrode to the client to hold firmly. The grip on the electrode should remain constant to prevent fluctuating current intensity to the follicle.
3 Apply anaphoresis if required.
4 Insert pre-sterilized needle into needle holder.
5 Probe follicle.
6 Treat test hair in chosen manner to determine blend setting.
7 When settings and balance of blend are established treat all hairs of similar type.
8 At the end of treatment cataphoresis may be applied. This has a number of advantages: use of the positive electrode has a germicidal effect by producing hydrochloric acid and restoring the skin's pH balance. Nerve endings are soothed which gives a feeling of well-being to the client. Erythema is reduced.
9 At the conclusion of the treatment, apply suitable aftercare.

## Body technique

The body technique allows the operator to work at a much faster rate by increasing the intensity of high frequency. To allow for the higher intensities, the time must be adjusted according to the client's pain threshold. The galvanic current flows constantly throughout the entire application to the follicle. However, the high frequency is pulsed at one-second intervals which reduces sensation.

## Current application and intensities during treatment

1 Set the high-frequency intensity according to the client's tolerance level.
2 Apply the high-frequency current for one second. Test to see if the hair will release. Repeat the procedure. If the hair is not easily removed after the second application, a further second of current may be given. Remove treated hairs manually if there is still traction after the third insertion.
3 Once the high-frequency setting and application time have been assessed, decide on the units of lye required for the type of hair being treated, in order to determine the galvanic milliamp setting, e.g.

> 3 seconds h/f divided into 45 u/l = 1.5 ma galvanic
> 3 seconds h/f divided into 60 u/l = 2.0 ma galvanic
> 4 seconds h/f divided into 60 u/l = 1.5 ma galvanic

There are a number of variations for current application when using body technique. With time and experience it will be possible to determine the most suitable method of application for each client.

In Figure 13.12 the galvanic current is applied to the follicle without interruption. The high frequency is pulsed at intervals of one second on and one second off. This has the effect of reducing discomfort to the client while the electrolysist can work at a higher speed. The technique is not to be recommended for the face. The application time and rest intervals can be varied according to the requirements of the individual. Machines offering the body technique facility are a great help when applying the currents in this manner.

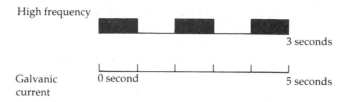

**Figure 13.12** Current application during standard body technique

High frequency

3 seconds

Galvanic current

0 second          5 seconds

It must be stressed that the body technique is not suitable for facial work. This is because the currents are set at a much higher intensity. Honey-coloured crusts appear on the surface of the skin after treatment, which may last up to three weeks. This is due to the increased chemical action that occurs as a result of the higher current settings. When the crusts fall off there is often a faint white mark left behind. Whereas this may be acceptable on the legs or body, the same reaction on the face would be undesirable.

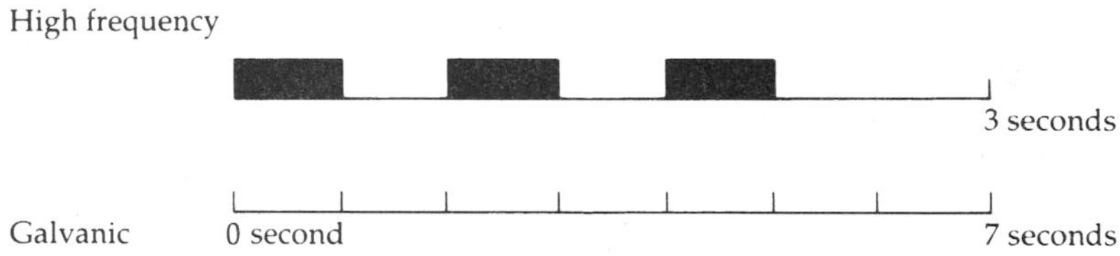

High frequency

3 seconds

**Figure 13.13** Current application, method A

Galvanic

0 second          7 seconds

Method B leads and finishes application with galvanic current only to enhance lye production.

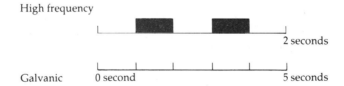

High frequency

2 seconds

**Figure 13.14** Current application, method B

Galvanic

0 second          5 seconds

# Progressive technique

The two-handed technique, also known as progressive epilation is the most effective way of destroying the follicle resulting in the minimum of regrowth. This is the preferred method in America, Canada, Holland and New Zealand. For many electrolysists who were trained in the one-handed technique used for shortwave diathermy the transition to the two-handed technique is far from easy. However it is worth persevering, for the results are far superior.

*Method of application – progressive ilepation*

Insert the needle into the hair follicle, then apply both currents. When the currents are flowing freely gently take hold of the hair with the tweezers without applying undue tension to the hair. After 4–6 seconds gently lift

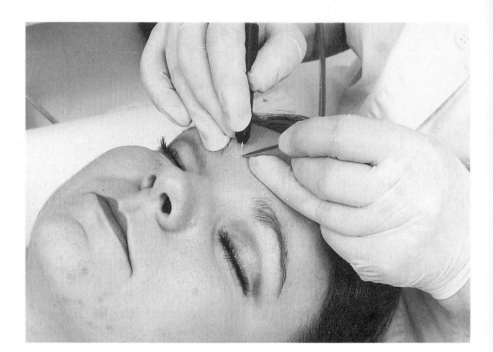

**Figure 13.15** Centre forehead, two-handed method, right-handed operator

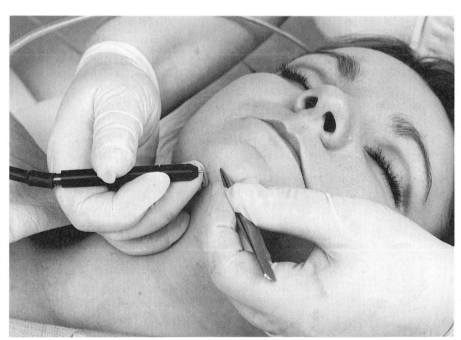

**Figure 13.16** Chin, two-handed method, right-handed operator

the hair and test for release. Test every few seconds until the hair releases. After the hair has been lifted from the follicle turn off the high frequency current only, keep the needle in the follicle and continue with 2–4 seconds of galvanic current. The additional lye created at this stage fills the follicle and ensures that all areas of the empty follicles are exposed to lye. At this

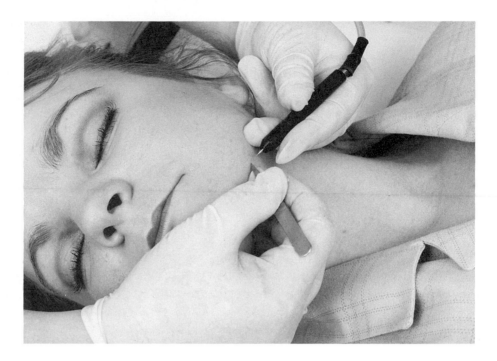

**Figure 13.17** Chin, two-handed method, left-handed operator

stage it will be possible to see lye froth appearing at the surface of the follicle.

Electrologists must take care not to touch the needle with the tweezers during the application of high frequency current. This action would result in a short circuit of the high frequency and prevents the current from entering the follicle.

Mistakes which often occur when first attempting progressive electrolysis are:

1 Taking hold of the hair with tweezers prior to needle insertion. This action may result in lifting the skin's surface and changing the direction of the follicle, so hindering correct and accurate insertion.
2 Touching the needle with the tweezers.
3 Applying continuous tension to the hair through current application. This action will result in the needle being inserted too deeply into the follicle. This will hinder the release of the hair from the follicle and will give insufficient treatment to the target area.

***Treatment procedure***

1 Remove any make-up or lipstick in the immediate area. Prepare and sanitize area to be treated.
2 Give the sponge-covered positive electrode to the client to hold firmly.
3 Examine the skin and hair and select the correct needle size, that is, match the diameter to the hair.
4 Insert pre-sterilized needle into needle holder.
5 Establish depth of insertion.
6 Determine working point, see pages 99 and 100, determining the balance of the blend and establishing the current setting for the blend.

7   Insert probe into follicle.
8   Gently hold hair with tweezers.
9   Progressively epilate.
10   Apply galvanic after-count to follicle.
11   At the conclusion of the treatment, apply suitable aftercare.

**Review questions**

1   What is meant by the 'blend'?
2   How does blend work?
3   Why is blend more versatile than either galvanic electrolysis or short-wave diathermy used independently?
4   Describe the action of the high-frequency current during blend application.
5   Describe the action of the galvanic current during blend application.
6   Why is the correct balance of the two currents important during blend application?
7   Explain the term 'lye'.
8   What is meant by the term 'units of lye'?
9   What determines the settings of the two currents during blend application?
10   Describe the two methods most widely used for establishing the current setting for blend.
11   Name the five variations of blend application.
12   Describe the treatment procedure for the blend.
13   How does the body technique work?
14   What is the purpose of body technique?
15   How does the body technique vary from general technique?
16   Why is it not advisable to use body technique on the face?

# 14 Practical application of electrical epilation

The question is often asked 'What is electrical epilation and why is it necessary?'

Quite simply, electrical epilation is the permanent removal of unwanted hair. This is brought about by the destruction of the lower hair follicle, through the application of an electrical current. The current used may be radio or high frequency, direct or galvanic, or a combination of the two currents referred to as *blend*.

**Who needs electrical epilation?**

Any person who has a problem with, or is embarrassed by, hair growth could well benefit from electro-epilation. It must be remembered that some problems occur as a result of an endocrine disorder, which could require medical treatment prior to electro-epilation treatment. Hair growth is a problem which affects any age range or social background.

The points to be considered when giving treatment are:

1  operator's posture and position during treatment;
2  positioning of client;
3  positioning of the equipment;
4  selection of needle size;
5  preparation of the area to be treated;
6  technique;
7  rhythm and continuity;
8  accuracy of probing;
9  current adjustment;
10  aftercare and homecare advice.

Should any one of the above not be carried out correctly there will be an adverse effect on the other areas, which in turn will have a detrimental effect on treatment.

**Operator's posture**

The correct posture is one that can be maintained with ease throughout the working day. There should be no undue fatigue or strain. The position of the back, shoulder, arm, wrist and hand should be considered in relation to the area being treated.

The back should be straight, with the body tilted slightly forward from the hips when necessary. The shoulders should be relaxed, muscles should not be tensed or raised towards the ears. When lifting or raising the arm, the shoulder should remain relaxed.

Arm, wrist and hand are kept in alignment with the follicle and direction of hair growth. This will help in achieving accurate insertions.

Incorrect posture will result in fatigue, backache and tightening of the shoulder muscles. This in turn could lead to a number of problems, including, in the long term, a frozen shoulder and/or consistent lower back problems, and in the short term severe headaches and/or painful neck and shoulders.

Standing for any length of time is not to be recommended. This position is tiring, prevents use of the foot switch and affects balance, which in turn will affect probing technique. It must be remembered that at times it will be necessary to stand for clients who need to be kept in an upright position, for example those with respiratory problems such as emphysema, or conditions such as hernia or vertigo.

Leaning on a client during treatment can be embarrassing and distasteful to the client, as well as uncomfortable.

## Operator's position

The correct working position during treatment should enable the operator to:

1  maintain correct posture;
2  align the probe to the direction of the hair growth, so aiding entry of the needle into the follicle;
3  reach the area requiring treatment easily.

To achieve this the operator must work on the *correct* side of the treatment couch. Right-handed operators work on the left side of the couch, whereas left-handed operators will work on the right side of the couch. Exceptions to this rule are illustrated on pages 116 and 117.

The operator's working position can be enhanced by the use of a stool or chair that is adjustable in height.

## Assessment of the client to prior to and during treatment

It is essential that the operator observes the client carefully both before and during treatment. The client's mood or sensitivity to treatment varies from one visit to another. Observe whether clients are relaxed or tense when they enter the treatment room, and whether they are tired or make reference to headaches or health problems etc.

During the treatment observe skin reaction, client's response and pain tolerance. Should the client tense during treatment, the current intensity should be reduced. When the client finds the treatment uncomfortable it is better to reduce the intensity and apply current for a little longer.

## Positioning of client

Clients should be positioned so that they are comfortable and relaxed, and so that undue embarrassment is avoided. At the same time the area requiring treatment should be easily accessible to the operator. Where there is a problem such as hiatus hernia, or where respiratory difficulties are present, it may be necessary to raise the client into a sitting position. When working on the upper lip it is important that the client's breathing is not hindered in any way.

Elderly clients and those with walking difficulties due to conditions such as arthritis and hip replacements may not be able to get onto the treatment couch easily. This should be taken into consideration and treatment procedure adjusted accordingly.

Clients in wheelchairs may need to receive treatment in their chair. In this instance it will be necessary to reposition the equipment and operator's stool accordingly. The operator should ensure that it is still possible to insert the needle easily and without causing skin damage.

***Preparation of electrologist's hands prior to treatment***

See Chapter 18, page 143.

# Positioning of equipment

The lamp should be placed so that the area is clearly lit, without causing shadows. When magnification is required the lens should be parallel to the area in order to avoid distortion of hairs. When positioned at the correct height the operator should be able to move the hands freely without knocking the lens. With fine vellus hairs it is often necessary to angle the light to the side, which will make the hairs easier to see.

The machine and trolley should be placed so that both are easily accessible during treatment. This will enable the operator to:

1   adjust the current when necessary without losing continuity;
2   see the machine easily;
3   reach accessories such as forceps, cotton wool and antiseptic easily.

Leads and cables from the equipment should be placed so that the risk of either client or operator tripping over them is minimized.

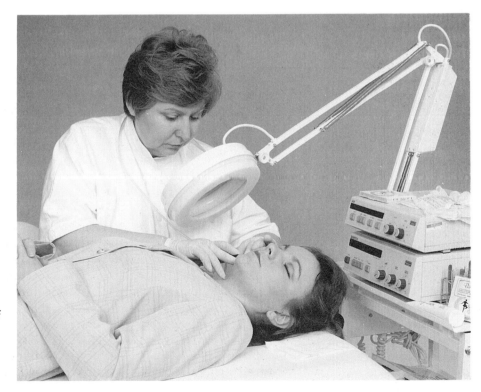

**Figure 14.1a** Position of right-handed operator in relation to couch, client and equipment when treating the face

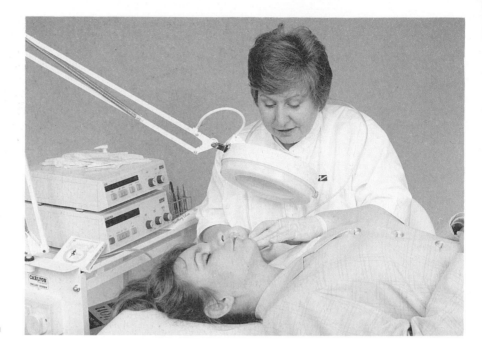

**Figure 14.1b** Position of left-handed operator in relation to couch, client and equipment when treating the face. Right-handed operators should be seated with the right side of their body next to the couch

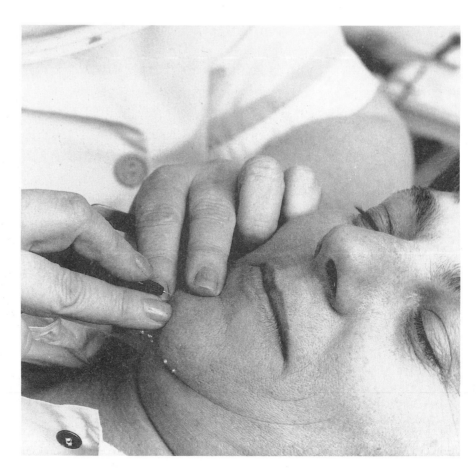

**Figure 14.1c** Point of chin. Right-handed operator

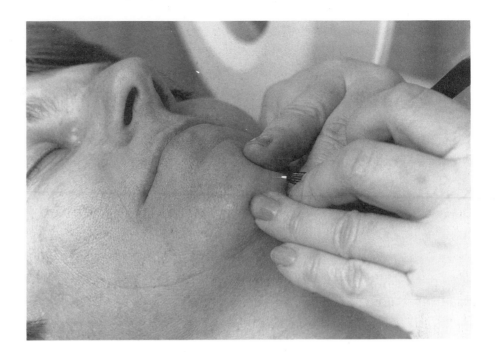

**Figure 14.1d** Point of chin. Left-handed operator

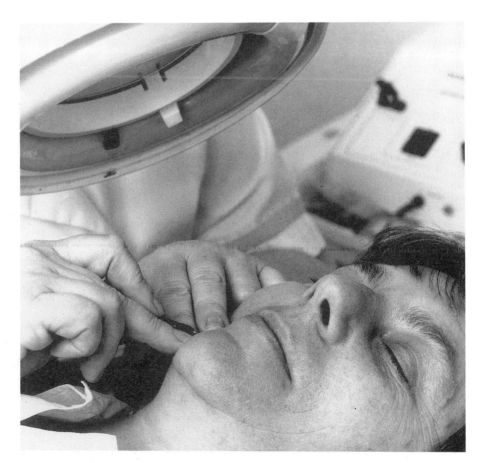

**Figure 14.1e** Side of chin. Right-handed operator

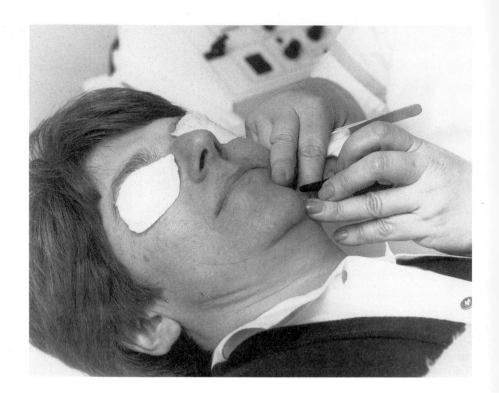

**Figure 14.1f** Side of chin. Left-handed operator

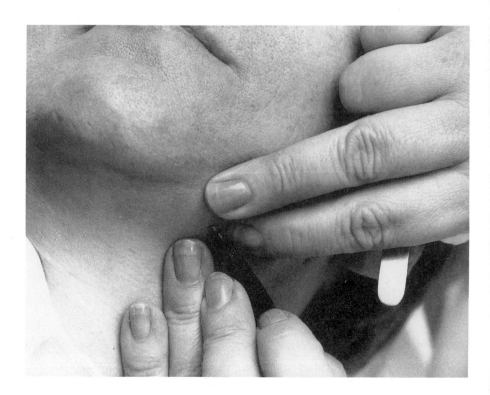

**Figure 14.1g** Left side of neck. Left-handed operator

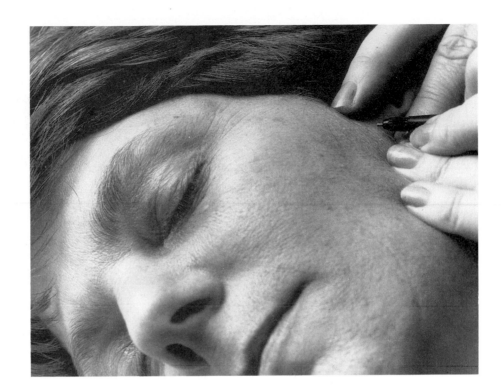

**Figure 14.1h** Side of face. Left-handed operator

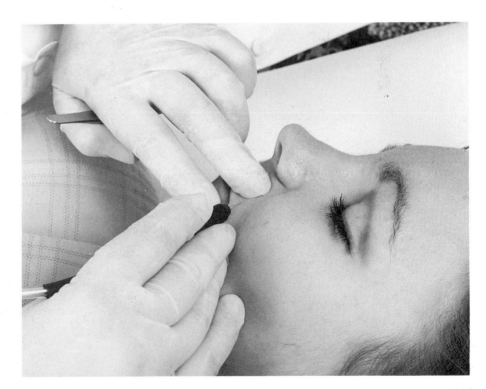

**Figure 14.1i** Upper lip. Right-handed operator

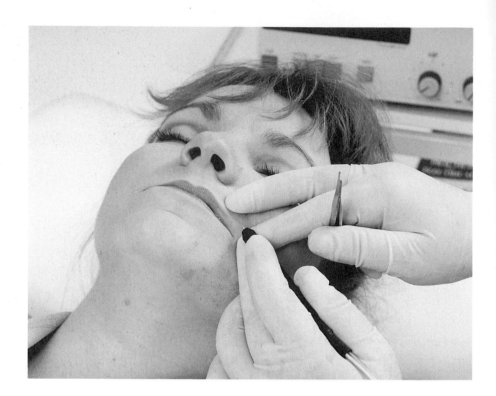

**Figure 14.1j** Upper lip. Left-handed operator

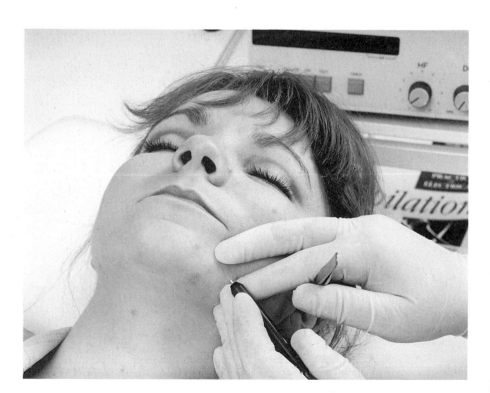

**Figure 14.1k** Side of jaw. Left-handed operator

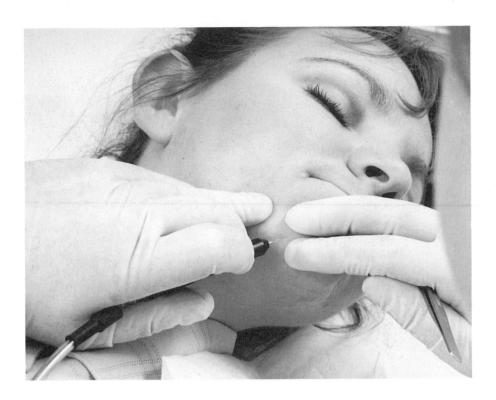

**Figure 14.1l** Side of jaw. Right-handed operator

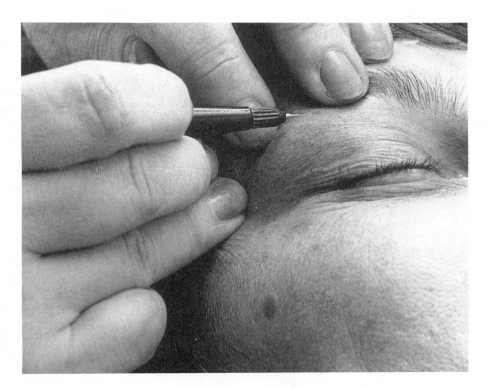

**Figure 14.1m** Eyebrows. Right-handed operator seated to the side of the treatment couch

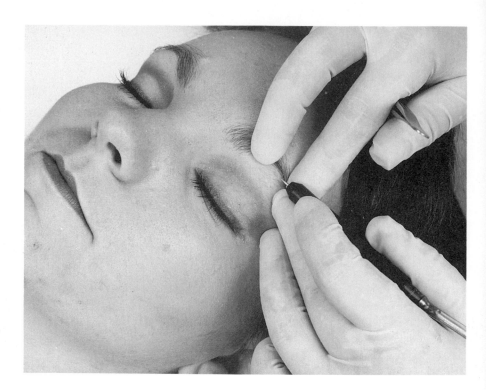

**Figure 14.1n** Eyebrows. Left-handed operator seated at head of couch

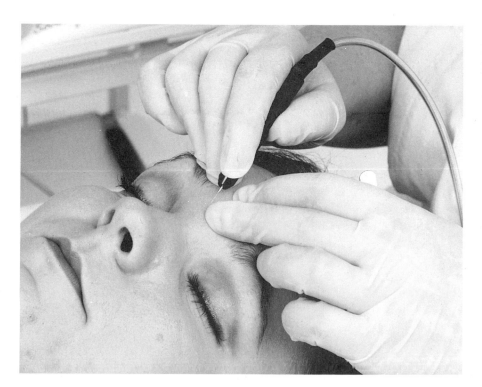

**Figure 14.1o** Centre eyebrows. Right-handed operator seated at head of couch

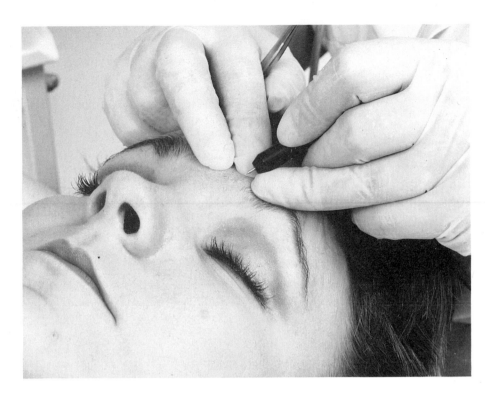

**Figure 14.1p** Centre eyebrows. Left-handed operator seated at head of couch

## Needle selection

The type and texture of the hair to be treated should be examined closely. The diameter of the needle chosen should correspond with the diameter of the hair. This will ensure that the needle tip is able to distribute sufficient current to the base of the follicle. A needle that is too large in diameter will stretch the follicle opening, which may result in bruising. There is also a risk of surface burns due to the needle being in contact with the skin at the follicle opening.

## Preparation of the area to be treated

Any make-up or lipstick in the immediate area should be removed thoroughly with a suitable cleanser. The skin to be treated should be wiped over with cotton wool and an antiseptic solution. Surgical spirit is not to be recommended – it has a drying effect on the skin, can be an irritant to sensitive skins, and is flammable.

## Technique

The stretch of the skin and the handling of the needle holder, needle and tweezers during insertion and removal of the hair all contribute to the efficiency of the treatment.

The skin should be held firmly but lightly. At no time should any undue weight or pressure be put on the skin during treatment. The stretch should open the follicle orifice to allow easy insertion of the needle without distorting the follicle in any way.

The hand holding the probe should rest very gently on the skin. The fingers of the opposite hand should be positioned in a manner which does not hinder the correct insertion of the needle.

## Probing technique

Accurate probing is essential if treatment is to be effective. The needle should enter the follicle easily, following the direction of hair growth. Slight resistance should be felt when the needle tip reaches the base of the follicle.

During probing, entry of the needle into the follicle should not be hindered by the fingers which stretch the skin. There should be no visible puckering or depression of the skin during insertion.

At no time should the needle be rotated in the follicle since this reduces the therapist's sensitivity and increases the risk of piercing the follicle wall.

Double depressions of either foot pedal or finger switch is not acceptable as normal practice. The need for double depressions indicates incorrect current intensity. The application of double depression using a finger switch increases the risk of forcing the needle through the base of the follicle on the second depression.

The finger switch should be depressed gently and smoothly. If the depression is too heavy the needle can be moved in the follicle so that it hits the wall of the follicle and pierces the base.

The angle of insertion should follow the direction of hair growth with the needle raised slightly from the skin's surface. There should be no loss of colour or depression in the skin through the needle leaning on the surface.

When the needle is resting or pressed on to the follicle wall surface burns can result. Incorrect angle of insertion could also result in the needle tip piercing the follicle wall or entering the sebaceous gland.

Insertions which are not deep enough and do not reach the base of the follicle may give rise to surface burns due to the current being applied too close to the epidermis. Insertions which are too deep result in destruction of the deeper tissue, eventually leaving pit marks in the skin where the tissue has collapsed.

The needle holder should be held very lightly and without tension.

When gripping the needle holder too tightly the operator's sensitivity during probing is lost.

The needle should slide smoothly into the follicle followed by application of current, withdrawal of needle and removal of hair. A correctly epilated hair should slide easily out of the follicle without signs of traction. The sequence should be smooth, rhythmic, but unhurried. Unnecessary hesitation during treatment wastes time and does not inspire the client with confidence.

## Current adjustment

Sufficient current should be used to destroy the hair follicle permanently without causing the client undue pain or adverse skin reaction. The current intensity is determined by the following factors:

1 type of hair;
2 skin sensitivity;
3 area being treated;
4 client's pain threshold.

**Figure 14.2** Position of the therapist (top) and client (bottom)

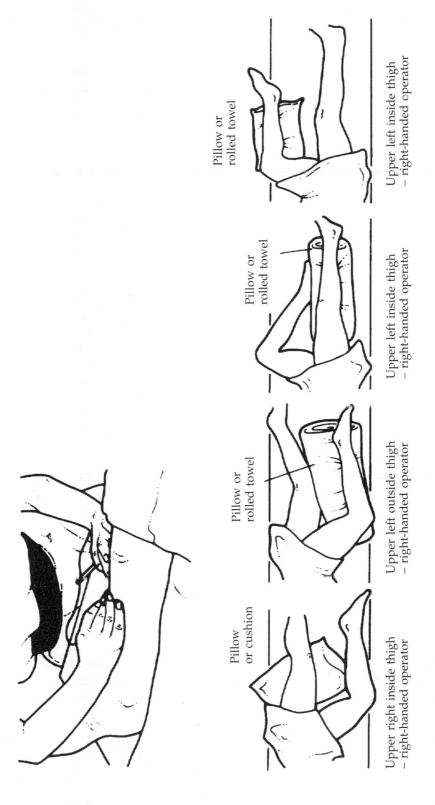

Pillow or rolled towel

Upper left inside thigh – right-handed operator

Pillow or rolled towel

Upper left inside thigh – right-handed operator

Pillow or rolled towel

Upper left outside thigh – right-handed operator

Pillow or cushion

Upper right inside thigh – right-handed operator

Position of client when treating upper leg

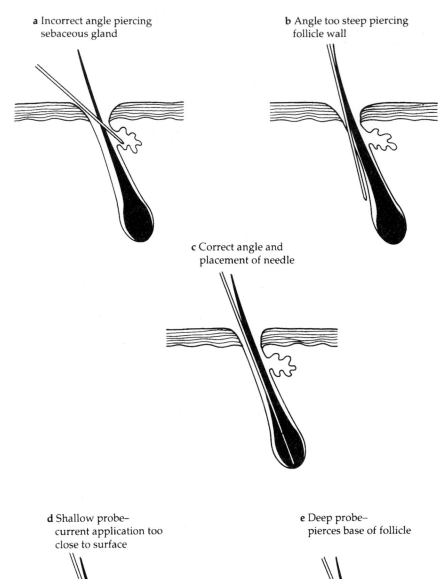

a Incorrect angle piercing sebaceous gland

b Angle too steep piercing follicle wall

c Correct angle and placement of needle

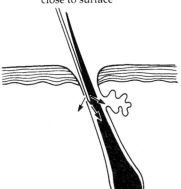

d Shallow probe–current application too close to surface

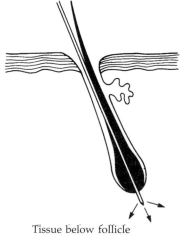

e Deep probe–pierces base of follicle

**Figure 14.3** Probing technique

Tissue destroyed too close to skin's surface

Tissue below follicle destroyed pit mark scar

**Figure 14.4** Position of correctly inserted needle in hair follicle

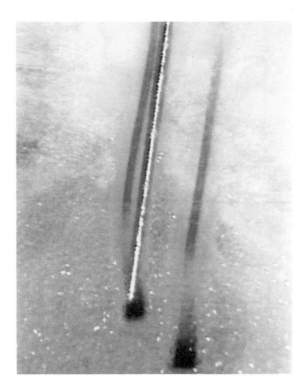

5 weather and atmospheric temperature, for example humidity and hot weather, bring about increased local circulation and more moisture in the skin. Therefore hairs may release easily with a lower current intensity;

6 when external temperature is cold the follicles close and nerve endings become more sensitive. This often results increased sensitivity and a lower pain threshold;

7 premenstrual tension and stress can also result in a lower pain threshold.

When the current is set to the correct intensity the hair will slide out of the follicle easily, complete with bulb, depending on the hair growth cycle. Dark terminal hairs on the chin will require a higher current intensity than fine terminal or vellus hairs on the upper lip. The client's pain threshold is much lower on the upper lip, particularly in the centre where the nerve endings are more numerous. A fine, sensitive skin will tolerate less current than a coarse or oily skin. See page 124 for details of skin types in relation to current.

Incorrect adjustment of current causes a number of problems. Too little current will result in under-treating of hair follicles with a higher percentage of regrowth than is acceptable. Too much current when using high frequency may result in over-treatment of skin, excess swelling, erythema, blanching and surface burns; too much current when using direct galvanic current may result in weeping follicles.

When the needle is too small a higher current intensity is needed in order to give enough current distribution to achieve follicle destruction.

The tweezers should be held in such a way that they do not scratch or irritate the client during probing. They should be easily accessible to the therapist during treatment so that continuity is not lost.

## Rhythm and continuity

There should be no 'stabbing' and no unnecessary selection of hairs. The treatment should be continuous without interruptions or unwarranted changes or adaptations to the routine. Check with the client to see which hairs are causing her most distress, then treat the strongest and/or most noticeable hairs first.

## Pain threshold

The skin has an abundant supply of sensory nerves contained within the dermis. Many fine fibrils or nerve endings reach up into the Malpighian layer of the epidermis. These are the sensory receptors of the skin which respond to heat, touch, cold, pain and pressure. The receptors which respond to pain are known as 'free nerve endings' (see Chapter 1).

The nerve supply around the hair follicle forms a fixed network. During late anagen the follicle grows down below the network, which is an advantage to the electrolysist. When the current is applied further away from the skin's surface, i.e. at the base of an anagen follicle, the sensory nerve endings take longer to respond.

Areas such as the upper lip react strongly to pain due to many nerve endings overlapping. Pain threshold varies from one area to another and from one individual to another. It is affected by stress, fatigue, anxiety, general health, and the menstrual cycle – particularly before and during the early stages of menstruation.

When work is concentrated on one area nerve fatigue will occur, numbing the nerve endings and lessening the sensation felt by the client. It is better therefore to work systematically in one area rather than to jump from one area to another.

The term 'pain threshold' refers to the amount of stimulation to free nerve endings that the individual can comfortably tolerate without drawing away from the source of pain. A low pain threshold means that the individual is able to tolerate only a low degree of stimulation.

## Treatment organization

The organization of treatment time needs to be efficient. The client will want to feel that she is being given value for money, so time must not be wasted. At the same time she must not feel that she is being rushed in and out of the treatment room as if she were on a conveyor belt. Nor must she feel that her money is all that the therapist is interested in.

During the session treat the darkest and most noticeable hairs first. Consult with the client to ascertain which hairs are causing her most concern. When the hair growth is dense it is advisable to treat every other hair. This will prevent over-treatment of the area and undue build-up of heat or sodium hydroxide. Allow sufficient healing space between hairs. Treat all hairs of a similar size and texture. Hair texture can range from fine to coarse in any one area. Therefore it may well be advisable to change the needle size during treatment. The importance of changing the needle size when necessary cannot be stressed sufficiently. The therapist should avoid touching the area that has just been treated.

## Aftercare and homecare advice

At the conclusion of treatment a soothing, medicated cream or lotion should be applied to the area. There are a number of suitable products available such as 'Witch Doctor' and 'Lacto Calamine'. Tinted aftercare preparations are also available for those clients who prefer to cover the erythema. The importance of correct aftercare must be explained to the client.

Clients should be advised not to apply make-up to the immediate area until the next day, at which time an aftercare cream should be applied to form a barrier between the skin and the make-up. Harsh soaps and perfumed products should be avoided. Similarly the client should be advised not to go swimming where there is a risk of picking up infection. Chlorine in the water will irritate the skin. Exposure to sunlight or sun beds creates heat on heat and therefore healing rate will be slower. There is also a possibility of pigmentation marks occurring. Tights, jeans or tight clothing should not be worn after treatment of the bikini line, in order to prevent friction.

## Length and frequency of treatment

The length of treatment sessions is determined by the density and texture of hair growth, the skin's sensitivity, the client's pain threshold and the size of the area to be treated.

The frequency of treatments will depend on the size of the area to be treated, the regrowth period and the time the client has available.

When treatments are too close together there may be insufficient hair to treat. More importantly the skin may not have had time to heal. When treatments are too far apart the results are slower. The hair growth cycle should be explained to the client so that the importance of attending for treatment regularly is understood.

Client psychology can also play a part in determining frequency of treatments. When a large area needs treatment, such as the legs, a client may prefer longer treatments to clear as much hair as possible in any one session. Where an area such as the lip, chin and sides of the face need attention, the areas can be worked in rotation so that the client can have several shorter treatments more frequently, yet still avoid working in any one area before sufficient healing time has elapsed. Psychologically the client feels better when attending more regularly.

## Management of hair growth between treatments

Many clients are worried about remaining hair growth after treatment. Due to the embarrassment, the majority of clients are not prepared to leave this hair alone. Therefore specific advice must be given by the therapist at the time of the consultation and reinforced after treatment.

The ideal is for the client to cut the hair, with scissors, close to the skin. This will not distort the follicle or affect the hair growth in any way.

When a large area is involved, shaving may be the most suitable alternative. However this can make the skin tender and will leave a shadow on the skin's surface as the hair grows.

## Effect of skin type on current application
*Dry skin*

This may be classified as either lacking sebum or lacking moisture. Skin with a low moisture content is referred to as dehydrated. Needle insertion may be hindered by dead skin cells blocking the follicle opening. Both high frequency and galvanic currents require moisture in order to work effectively.

**Oily skin**

Here there is a surface covering of sebum which acts as an excellent insulator. This has the advantage of confining the current to the lower follicle where it is needed. The moisture content of the lower follicle is usually good. Due to the presence of open pores, needle insertion is relatively easy. Comedones, papules or pustules may be present. The skin texture is often thicker than that of normal or dry skin. The pH balance of oily skin may be disturbed, which increases the risk of infection.

**Moist skin**

Moist skin has a high moisture content within both the dermis and epidermis, therefore considerable care should be taken during current application. There is a risk of high-frequency action rising up the follicle too quickly and reaching the skin's surface before the lower follicle has been successfully treated. Blend is possibly more suitable for this skin type because a lower intensity of high frequency is used. The galvanic action will occur relatively quickly.

**Sensitive skin**

This is often fine in texture with telangiectasia (red capillaries). This type of skin may be dry or oily and reacts quickly to the heat produced by high frequency. Sensitive skin often responds well to blend, particularly when phoresis is applied either before and/or after treatment.

## Assessing the skin's appearance during treatment

Loss of colour around the follicle during insertion may be due to using a needle which is too large, or to the operator leaning the needle on the skin.

Loss of colour during galvanic action is the result of gas and sodium hydroxide building up under the skin's surface during treatment.

Gas vapour may appear on one side of the needle during galvanic treatment, but may also result from a combination of moisture and hydrogen gas when blend is applied.

A blue or black lump indicates bruising from incorrect probing, which pierces or damages the capillaries. Immediate pressure should be applied with dry sterile cotton wool or a cold compress.

Blanching of the skin during high-frequency treatment occurs when the currency is too high or is applied too close to the surface.

Weeping follicles shortly after treatment are an indication that too much galvanic current has been used, resulting in excessive chemical decomposition of the skin tissues.

**Evaluating hair regrowth**

Hair regrowth should be monitored carefully. Sometimes a client will comment that the hairs reappear within a few days of treatment. There are two reasons for this:

1 Hairs were not epilated correctly. True regrowth appears from follicles which have not received sufficient current or through inaccurate insertions which have missed the lower follicle and dermal papilla.
2 Hairs are entirely different hairs to those which have previously been treated. At this stage it is advisable to go through a brief explanation of the hair growth cycle. Clients who have just started a course of epilation treatment and who have been plucking for some time are often shocked to realize how many hairs need treatment. Due to the fact that plucking/tweezing has been carried out on a regular basis the individual is unaware of the extent of the problem.

**Incorrect working techniques**

Incorrect working habits and poor techniques lead to an inefficient treatment and in many instances the formation of scars.

Apart from immediate post-epilation erythema and, of course, the fact that the hair growth is either considerably reduced or no longer present there should be no visible signs that treatment has taken place.

Blood spots, pinpricks and scabs are all undesirable after treatment with the exception of the formation of scabs on the body or legs when either blend body technique or high-frequency flash technique have been used.

*Habits to be avoided*

1 Stroking the hair or skin and undue hesitation between insertions leads to an inefficient treatment. Loss of rhythm and continuity could affect the client's confidence in the operator's ability.
2 The hair should not be lifted or rotated around the needle before insertion. This may lead to incorrect angle of insertion and consequently inefficient removal of hairs.
3 Incorrect posture of the operator is not only tiring over a period of time but also leads to faulty probing technique.
4 A tense or rigid hand and wrist during probing results in loss of operator sensitivity, and therefore the inability to sense the base of the follicle during needle insertion.
5 Holding the hair with tweezers before and during insertion distorts the follicle, which will alter the follicle angle and prevent smooth insertions.
6 Double depressions, which give two bursts of current to the follicle during a single insertion, are not recommended. The second depression can easily move the needle, which may then pierce the base of the follicle or move the needle on to the follicle wall. This can lead to incorrect current distribution and consequently to the formation of scars. This habit leads to excess current application and indicates incorrect current intensity.

**Causes of scarring**

1 Entering follicle with high frequency current on.
2 Coming out of the follicle with high-frequency current on.
3 Probing through the base of the follicle with the current on will result in destruction of lower tissues, eventually giving rise to a depression or pit mark on the surface of the skin.
4 Probing through the side of the follicle wall with the current on will also lead to pit marks and depressions, due to current being concentrated in the wrong area.
5 Shallow probing allows the application of high-frequency current too close to the skin's surface. Pigmentation marks will occur.
6 When high frequency current is applied for too long, too much heat will be produced. When application time of galvanic current is excessive too much sodium hydroxide will be produced.
7 Re-entering and applying current to the same follicle too often.
8 Over-treating area. When too many hairs are treated in a concentrated area, either too much heat will be produced by high frequency, giving rise to tissue damage, or there will be too much galvanic action, which will produce weeping follicles. There is also a risk of post-treatment infection.

9 When the intensity of current is too high with high frequency, excess heat is produced in the area. With galvanic current too much sodium hydroxide will occur.

10 A needle that is too large stretches the follicle wall, causing bruising, and may damage surface capillaries. Current dissipates at the skin's surface where the needle touches the follicle wall, so causing a surface burn.

11 The giving of treatment too often in the same area does not allow the deeper skin tissues to heal.

12 Poor-quality needles with rough surfaces, blunt or broken tips, may puncture the skin or give inefficient current distribution.

The following points are not direct causes of scarring but they might affect treatment and are therefore unacceptable:

1 When the skin is stretched incorrectly, accurate insertion is hindered or prevented.

2 Inaccurate position of hand and wrist results in the wrong angle and direction of needle entry into the follicle.

3 Lack of attention to aftercare may give rise to infection, chlorine in the water when swimming may set up an adverse skin reaction, sunbathing gives rise to heat on heat, which leaves the skin feeling tender. Applying make-up blocks the pores and fingering the area allows entry of bacteria.

4 Incorrect position/angle of lamp casts a shadow over the area to be treated.

## Advantages of electrical epilation over temporary methods

Electrical epilation, whether it is by blend, galvanic electrolysis or short-wave diathermy is the only permanent method of destroying hair.

There are a number of temporary methods, each of which has particular disadvantages, but the main disadvantage, common to all, is that the hair grows again.

*Chemical depilatories* remove the hair just below the skin's surface. They work by dissolving the hairs, and often the stratum corneum. The skin can become irritated and sensitive. An allergic reaction is common. Due to the removal of the stratum corneum, the skin's protective function is reduced, thereby increasing the risk of infection. Regrowth appears within two to five days.

*Plucking/tweezing* distorts the hair follicle. The hair growth is encouraged through stimulation of the local blood supply to the follicle base. Fine hairs can accidentally be removed. These may be stimulated into stronger growth, due to sensitivity of the follicle to circulating hormones within the blood. Clients are often tempted to pluck a few stray hairs as they appear. The skin is easily bruised by persistent or heavy-handed use of the tweezers.

Mechanical epilators have a similar effect to plucking. They rip the hair out by the root, distort the follicle and can be painful.

*Sugaring* dates back to the era of Anthony and Cleopatra, but is a relatively new concept in Britain. The principle of sugaring is similar to that of waxing. The sugaring substance is applied to the skin, then worked on to the hair and skin with the fingers. The product is then ripped off the skin with a lifting motion, which removes the hair by the root. Regrowth appears between three and six weeks later.

*Waxing* also removes the complete hair root when skilfully carried out. The drawback with waxing is that hairs are often broken off at the skin's surface, due to incorrect technique. Follicles become distorted. The regrowth period is between three and six weeks.

Both waxing and sugaring of facial hair can encourage the development of stronger regrowth of fine hairs. Ingrowing hairs often occur when using either of these methods.

On balance, it can be seen that although electrical epilation is slow, in the right hands it is both safe and effective.

## Record cards

Record cards should contain details of treatments, for example date of treatment, length of session, needle size, current intensity, area treated, skin reaction and electrologist's initials.

Accurate and well-maintained records enable the electrologist to keep track of the treatment, note progress or any changes in hair growth pattern which occurs.

## Equipment fails to work

There are times when equipment fails to work properly, often at the beginning of or during a treatment. When this happens the following procedure should be followed:

1 Epilation machine – check the needle holder to see if the lead is attached firmly. In many instances the lead may be broken in one of three places.
   (a) where the lead connects with the needle holder;
   (b) where the lead connects with the machine or;
   (c) a break in the lead somewhere in the middle.
2 If there is no light showing on the machine check the fuse in the plug and if necessary in the machine. (On receiving new equipment it is advisable to find out where the fuse is situated.)
3 Check that the wires to the plug are connected. Sometimes with continuous use one or more of the wires works loose.
4 When the magnifying lamp is not working try changing the bulb first. If this is not successful look at the starter unit situated near the bulb, this may need changing. The plug should also be checked as in 3 above.

## Review questions

1 List the factors that influence the successful and efficient application of electrical epilation.
2 Explain the effect of the electrolysist's posture on probing technique.
3 Why is it essential for the electrolysist to work from the correct side of the treatment couch?
4 State the factors that influence the positioning of equipment.
5 What is the purpose of stretching the skin while probing?
6 Explain the disadvantage of double depression of the button during current application
7 How can the electrolysist prove that the depth and angle of insertion during probing is correct?
8 Explain the effects on the skin and follicle of:

(a) shallow insertions;

(b) deep insertions.

9 What factors determine current intensity and current adjustment during treatment?

10 Explain the meaning of 'pain threshold'.

11 State the factors that influence the frequency and length of treatments.

12 List the considerations to be taken into account when deciding which hairs to treat during a session.

13 State the advice that should be given to clients in relation to aftercare at home.

14 Describe the most effective way for clients to manage hairgrowth in between appointments.

15 List the effects of the following on current application:

(a) moist skin

(b) dry skin

(c) oily skin.

16 Name and describe five working habits that could have an adverse effect on treatment.

17 Name and describe any seven causes of scarring.

18 What effect do chemical depilatories have on the hair and skin?

19 Why are clients discouraged from plucking hairs once a course of electrical epilation has begun?

20 Why is it acceptable for clients to wax or sugar the legs but not the face?

21 What is the advantage of electrical epilation over other methods of hair removal?

# 15 Consultation

The consultation provides a golden opportunity for a link to form between the electrolysist and the client. In many instances a great deal of courage is required for the client to make the initial appointment, and further courage is needed for them to walk through the clinic door. The electrolysist's approach at this stage will either encourage or discourage the potential client.

What are clients looking for during this initial contact with the electrolysist? Usually they are seeking a professional approach which is warm and welcoming – one that is not patronizing or that makes them feel abnormal or inferior. Questions may arise relating to the professional qualifications of the electrolysist, knowledge of the subject, frequency and length of treatments, time taken to clear the problem permanently, methods of dealing with the hair growth between appointments, cost involved, approach to hygiene, and the use of sterile disposable needles.

Having considered the advantages to the client, some thought should be given to the benefits of the consultation to the electrolysist. Valuable information can be obtained at this stage which will enable the electrolysist to plan an effective course of treatment. Several factors need to be considered before a decision on treatment is reached:

**Hair**

- Type of hair growth: fine, vellus, terminal, curly, straight
- Density and site of hair growth: chin, upper lip, body, bikini area
- Previous methods of hair removal: waxing, plucking, shaving, depilatory creams, cutting

The reason for discussing previous hair growth control and the frequency with which a particular method has been used is to establish whether follicles may have become distorted due to waxing or plucking. If this is the case then treatment with the blend may be more effective than shortwave diathermy, due to the inability to place the needle accurately at the base of the follicle. When the client has been plucking hair regularly she often does not realize the full extent of the problem, which may come as a shock once the tweezers have been banished!

Scarring may be present from electrical epilation received elsewhere. If so, type and extent should be noted, as should the length of time during which scarring has been evident.

**Skin**

Several points need to be looked at here: whether the skin is fine in texture or coarse, dry, oily or sensitive; the healing rate; and the presence of acne, infection, eczema, psoriasis or other skin conditions in the area to be treated. Does the client have any allergies to certain preparations or metals?

**Medical history**

At this stage a detailed medical history should be taken which must include the following:

- Possible contra-indications such as asthma and emphysema (see pages 134–5).
- Prescribed medications to include steroids, hormones, hormone replacement therapy, contraceptive pill, insulin, anti-coagulants, anti-depressants, tranquillizers, drugs for the control of epilepsy.
- Pregnancy: stage and any complications which may have arisen during the pregnancy.
- Hepatitis B: date of illness, prescribed drugs. (Notification of proposed treatment to doctor).
- Hepatitis C.
- Diabetes: whether controlled by diet, tablets or insulin injections. Healing rate and sensitivity of skin should be noted.
- Epilepsy: severity and frequency of attacks. Medication used.
- Circulatory disorders: to include any heart problems.
- Endocrine and gynaecological problems: polycystic ovary syndrome, menstrual irregularities, menopause, endometriosis.
- Surgery: date and nature.

Why is it necessary to obtain the above information, and how can it be of use in treatment planning? Most importantly, it enables the electrolysist to assess whether or not the treatment is right for the client. Is there a condition such as diabetes which requires liaison with the GP prior to the commencement of any treatment? With conditions such as polycystic ovary syndrome, medical treatment is required since without this, complete elimination is not possible.

During the menopause it is possible that hair growth will increase due to the change in the hormone balance. Some follicles become sensitive to these circulating hormones in the blood, and hair growth is stimulated. This can and does cause embarrassment.

A woman can become more sensitive with a lowered pain threshold immediately before and during menstruation, therefore the treatment will often be painful at this time. The skin can also take longer to heal.

During pregnancy there is an alteration in hormone levels and in a number of instances hair growth increases. This growth is often temporary and disappears after the birth of the baby without any form of treatment. There is no known reason why treatment to an existing problem should stop during the pregnancy but it is advisable to notify the client's GP of the treatment details.

Certain medications stimulate hair growth, e.g. steroids and some forms of hormone replacement, whereas others increase the risk of pigmentation, e.g. the contraceptive pill and those hormones used in large doses for transsexual clients.

Diabetic conditions require liaison with the GP and consideration should be given to the fact that skin is slower to heal, therefore treatment sessions should be spaced further apart. The pain threshold is also lower, particularly before a meal, due to the drop in blood-sugar level, and so timing of appointments needs to be carefully planned.

Should scars be present from previous electrical epilation treatment it is essential that these are pointed out to the client, as tactfully as possible, during the consultation. This will prevent any confusion at a later date as to the length of time during which the scars have been evident. In other words it will protect the electrolysist who gives further treatment.

At this stage a short explanation of the hair growth cycle helps the client to understand what is happening below the skin's surface and the importance of attending for treatment on a regular basis. The removal of a few hairs will enable the client to see how the treatment feels, while giving the electrolysist an opportunity to assess skin reaction. A simple description of how electrical epilation works will give the client an insight into why it is not possible to guarantee the destruction of any one hair permanently after a single treatment.

No consultation would be complete without the therapist examining the skin, preferably with the aid of a magnifying light. The colour and condition of the skin often gives an indication as to the health of the client, for example the colour may be high; there may be dilated capillaries, veins may be red or blue. If redness is in a butterfly pattern across nose and cheeks, rosacea may be indicated. Should the colour be blue there could be a respiratory or heart problem present.

A dull-grey appearance could indicate a smoker – oxygen supply to the skin will be affected due to the constricting effect of nicotine on the small blood vessels; this in turn will affect the healing rate of the skin. A yellow tinge to the skin could indicate a problem with either the gall bladder or the liver – with liver diseases there is often a tendency to develop spider naevi. A thin skin with a tendency to redness and sensitivity could be the result of steroid application.

Next, look at the condition and type of skin, e.g. is the skin oily with comedones, is it dry through lack of sebum, or dehydrated through lack of moisture? Does the skin bruise easily? Are there any pigmentation marks? If so, query the possible causes, e.g. medication, contraceptive pill. Is the texture coarse, thick, thin or fine? Are there signs of conditions such as eczema, psoriasis, acne?

The electrolysist should now be able to advise the client on the frequency of appointments, length of each session and cost per visit. It is usually not possible, or advisable, to give a time of completion concerning the permanent elimination of the problem.

There are rare occasions when a prospective client will be reluctant to give the electrologist information relating to medical history and previous treatment during a consultation. This type of client can be difficult to treat. Explain to the client why the information is needed. Quite often by going through the different questions with an explanation of why they are being asked the client will respond with a negative or positive answer, for example, 'that doesn't apply to me', or 'I am not taking hormone replacement or medication'. In this way it is sometimes possible to gain the relevant information. When the prospective client refuses to answer questions relating to medical history and will not allow you to contact a general practitioner then it would not be wise to proceed with the treatment.

Alternatively continue the consultation without pursuing the matter of medical history. Give a detailed explanation of electrolysis and how it works. Then give the prospective client a leaflet which explains what electrolysis is and how it works. (These are available from specialist professional associations.) Suggest that the prospective client goes home to give the matter further thought before undertaking treatment.

## Assessing the client

Is the client calm and confident or nervous, agitated, embarrassed, or on the defensive or attack? What is the client's life-style? Does she have the time to attend for treatment on a regular basis? Is she prepared to follow instructions for aftercare and management of hair growth between treatments?

During the consultation the electrolysist should take the opportunity to enquire how the client came to hear about the clinic/electrolysist. Was it by recommendation, through a professional association, advertising or passing by?

When conducted thoroughly, the consultation gives the electrolysist a comprehensive picture of the new client and her needs. Any contra-indications which may be present (see pages 134 and 135) should be observed at this time, and an explanation given to the client as to why treatment with electrical epilation is not to be recommended. The client should be placed under no obligation to proceed with treatment should she not wish to do so. When a consultation has been conducted in the right manner with the correct professional approach, there are very few clients who leave the clinic without making a further appointment.

## The effects of unwanted hair growth on a client's psychology

The presence of unwanted hair growth usually has a demoralizing effect on a woman, resulting in loss of self-confidence. The individual may show signs of being inhibited, shy, aggressive, argumentative or defensive in order to mask her feelings of embarrassment. The electrolysist should be able to read the body language displayed by the prospective client in order to assess the best method of approach. For many individuals a great deal of courage is required to pick up the telephone and make an appointment. Even more courage is needed to walk through the clinic door at the scheduled time. The electrolysist's manner and approach at the initial meeting is of vital importance.

The author never fails to be pleasantly surprised by the personality changes that take place in many clients once a course of treatment has been started. Shy, inhibited individuals become more outgoing and interested in life in general. Aggressive, argumentative and defensive traits disappear. The client becomes more confident and relaxed and the hair growth problem becomes less of a dominant factor in her life. A statement made by many clients is 'electro-epilation has changed my life. I feel a different person and so much happier'. These personality changes are due to the sympathy, understanding and professional manner of the electrolysist, in combination with the successful results of electro-epilation treatment.

## Client's expectations of treatment

During the initial consultation it is helpful to find out what the client's expectations of treatment are. In many instances the prospective client is under the impression that hair removal will be permanent after the first electrolysis treatment. Often they have read misleading advertisements or read articles in magazines or local papers.

It is at this stage that the prospective client should be given a clear understanding as to the role of electrolysis and that for best results a commitment should be made by the client to follow the treatment plan and advice on hair control recommended by the electrologist.

It is important to ensure that the client understands that the hair growth did not occur overnight and therefore it will not disappear overnight. Electrolysis is a progressive treatment which will achieve results in the end. An explanation of the hair growth cycle during the consultation will help the client to have a clearer understanding of why there sometimes appears to be instant regrowth after treatment and why the problem can not be cleared overnight.

**Review questions**

1 List the advantages of the initial consultation to the client.
2 List the advantages of the initial consultation to the electrolysist.
3 Why is it necessary to discuss previous hair growth control?
4 What details should be taken relating to medical history?
5 State the advantage of explaining the hair growth cycle to the client.
6 What should the electrolysist look for while examining the client's skin?
7 State the information that can be obtained from assessing the client during a consultation.
8 Explain the psychological effect on a client of unwanted hair growth.

# 16 Contra-indications

There are a number of conditions that are either contra-indicative – i.e. show that treatment is inadvisable or dangerous, or that require advice from the client's doctor prior to commencement of electro-epilation.

- Asthma: defined as 'a condition characterized by transient narrowing of the smaller airways'. During an asthmatic attack the patient experiences great difficulty in breathing. May be triggered by anxiety or stress. Should the client's GP agree to electro-epilation treatment, particular attention should be given to positioning during the session.
- Dermagraphic skin condition: congenital sensitivity to any form of friction on the skin. Swelling appears shortly after treatment and may last up to 24 hours. No long-term adverse effects, but the decision concerning continuation of treatment should be the client's.
- Dermatitis/eczema in area: increased sensitivity, skin irritated and often a build-up of dry skin blocks opening to follicle thereby hindering insertion.
- Fungal infections, e.g. tinea: risk of transmitting infection.
- Bacterial infections, e.g. impetigo: risk of transmitting infection.
- Viral infections, e.g. herpes simplex, herpes zoster: risk of cross-infection.
- Heart problems/circulatory disorders requiring medical treatment: advisable to consult with GP.
- Haemorrhage/bruising: disturbed blood supply interferes with healing process. Heating effect of shortwave diathermy causes blood vessels to dilate.
- Hypertension/anxiety, stress: nerve endings highly sensitive, client unable to relax therefore treatment more painful. Insertion to follicle hindered. Risk of scarring due to client pulling away during current application.
- Loss of skin sensation: inability to sense when current is too high, which could result in over treatment of area.
- Metal plate: concentration of high-frequency field causes overheating in tissues.
- Pre-malignant/malignant lesions: possible stimulation of metabolism due to increase in temperature could accelerate growth.
- Hepatitis C.

An additional consideration when using galvanic or blend treatments is the presence of excessive fillings which often give rise to a metallic taste in the mouth and which may be unacceptable to the client.

**Conditions which require liaison with the GP prior to treatment**

- Epilepsy: electrical impulses to brain may be disturbed which could result in a fit. Shortwave diathermy only should be given, particularly if anxiety is present.
- Vascular disorders requiring anti-coagulant drugs: coagulation of blood supply at base of follicle is hindered.
- Hepatitis B: use of gloves by operator is advisable. Strict attention to

hygiene and the use of disposable sterile needles is essential. The clotting mechanism is often affected, and the healing rate of the skin is inhibited. The client bruises easily.

- Naevi/moles: hairs growing out of moles must be referred to a general practitioner for check on possible malignancy.
- Diabetic condition: slow to heal, low pain threshold, shorter treatments, larger healing gaps, increased length of time between treatment sessions.
- Endocrine disorders: several endocrine disorders such as polycystic ovary syndrome result in increased hair growth in a male pattern. It is essential that correct medical treatment is carried out, which may aid in the reduction of unwanted hair. However it is worth remembering that electrical epilation in conjunction with medical treatment will speed up the final result.
- Emphysema: some drugs used in the control of emphysema can lead to an increase in hair growth. In extreme cases it may be possible only to keep the hair growth under control rather than to eliminate it. However it must be remembered that psychologically the electrical epilation may be of value to the client. Consideration must be given to the positioning of the client during treatment due to breathing difficulties.
- Steroids: often instrumental in encouraging hair growth.
- Hiatus hernia: positioning during treatment is of the utmost importance. The client should be raised to prevent discomfort.

**Review questions**

1 Define the term contra-indication.
2 Why are the following termed contra-indications to electrical epilation?
   (a) asthma;
   (b) herpes simplex;
   (c) loss of skin sensation.
3 Explain why it is necessary to liaise with the client's doctor when the following conditions exist:
   (a) epilepsy;
   (b) hairy moles;
   (c) endocrine disorders.
4 What complications arise from emphysema?

# 17 Advanced electrical epilation

Treatment of telangiectasia, warts and skin tags should only be undertaken by well-trained and fully experienced operators. It takes time to develop the sensitivity in the hands which is essential when performing advanced work.

**Telangiectasia**

This condition is more commonly referred to as broken veins, dilated capillaries, red veins, or thread veins. The correct terminology is telangiectasia, which refers to the dilation of small blood vessels in the skin.

This condition causes distress to many people of both sexes. However treatment by shortwave diathermy is possible in many instances. There are a number of reasons why telangiectasia develop. Investigation into the possible cause must take place prior to treatment.

*Causes/aggravating factors*

- *Asthma:* due to the transient narrowing of the air passages oxygen supply to the skin is impaired. Capillaries with a reddish/blue colour appear on the cheeks and around the nose.
- *Circulatory disorders* which result in weakened capillary walls. Certain medications may aggravate the condition.
- *Comedone extraction:* the repeated extraction of comedones, particularly around the nose, with too much pressure from fingernails, often damages the capillaries.
- *Diabetes:* the skin is both sensitive and dry. The blood is slow to coagulate and the skin bruises easily.
- *Diet:* certain foods such as hot curries and spicy foods are very stimulating. Alcohol causes the capillaries to dilate, as do very hot beverages such as tea and coffee. When drinks are too hot the heat from the steam raises the local temperature of the skin. Tea and coffee both contain the stimulant caffeine. Eating food too quickly also encourages the development of telangiectasia.
- *Hormones:* hyper-pigmentation of the skin and sensitivity to natural sunlight and sunbeds often occurs as a result of taking the contraceptive pill. There is a tendency for dilated capillaries to occur with increased skin sensitivity.
- *Pregnancy:* spider naevi often occur during pregnancy. If left untreated these will often disappear within six months of the birth. Small, blue veins appearing on the legs during pregnancy do not disappear. Unfortunately due to the depth of the feeder veins treatment of the legs is very rarely successful for any length of time. A long and strenuous labour can often aggravate existing facial telangiectasia.

- *Heredity:* hereditary disposition comes high on the list of causes. When questioned clients often refer only to the mother's history, overlooking the fact that skin problems can be inherited from the father and his predecessors!
- *Liver diseases:* the skin tends to develop spider naevi, telangiectasia and haemangiomas in abundance on the trunk of the body. Other areas such as the face and arms can be affected. The skin bruises easily.
- *Knocks/heavy blows:* such as those caused by bumping into the corner of an office desk may often cause dilated capillaries to occur.
- *Medications:* the application of steroid-based creams such as Betnovate thin the skin when used over a prolonged period of time, or when used too often. Increased redness, skin sensitivity and a tendency to develop telangiectasia are some of the side-effects of steroid creams. Antibiotics may cause an increase in spider naevi. Antihistamines dehydrate the skin, which also becomes sensitive to sunlight.
- *Extremes of temperature:* this can include frequent use of the steam bath and sauna – particularly if a cold shower is taken afterwards. Hot baths where the hot tap is left running are also not good for the skin due to the excessive heat. Long hours spent in a hot, steamy kitchen have a detrimental effect on facial capillaries. When the skin is subjected to any of the above on a regular basis, weak capillaries lose the ability to dilate and contract efficiently, eventually remaining in a state of constant dilation.
- *Tight clothing/pop socks:* restrict the circulation which puts pressure on the surface capillaries.
- *Respiratory problems:* these include asthma, hay fever and sinus problems. During the height of the hay fever season consistent sneezing tends to rupture the capillary walls. The skin is often sensitive.
- *Rosacea:* can vary from mild to severe forms. Telangiectasia first appear on the nose and cheeks in a butterfly appearance. As the condition progresses the skin texture thickens, papules form and the high colour intensifies. The colour can vary from pale pink in the early stages to a deep red with a blue tinge during the later stages. Medical control is usually by the administration of tetracycline.
- *Sensitivity:* to foods, harsh cosmetic preparations, incorrect skin care, e.g. too many facial scrubs, or over-stimulating face masks, and exposure to extremes of weather conditions. Sensitive skins have a tendency to flush easily. The continual dilation and contraction of capillaries can result in weakening of the capillary walls.
- *Spectacles:* with badly fitting frames and/or heavy glass lenses can put pressure on the bridge and sides of the nose as well as along the upper cheek bones. This encourages the development of telangiectasia where there is a weakness in the capillaries. Unless the cause is rectified the problem will recur in a very short period of time.
- *Smoking:* reduces the oxygen supply to the skin. Therefore cellular regeneration is decreased and the skin is slower to heal. A smoker's skin often has a grey, sluggish, dehydrated appearance. Fine lines can be seen, particularly around the mouth.
- *Sporting activities:* such as horse riding, high-powered speed boats, skiing

and water skiing may all result in the development of dilated capillaries. Any sport which involves frequent exposure to the elements, particularly at speed, will have a detrimental effect on the skin. Biting winds will cause windburn, reflection of ultraviolet rays from the snow can result in sunburn, and each will encourage the development of telangiectasia.

- *Sunlight:* in moderation has a beneficial effect on the skin. However over-exposure to the sun's rays or incorrect use of sunbeds causes a number of problems. Tissue fibres are weakened; dehydration of the skin occurs; sunburn and/or prolonged exposure to the sun damages the surface capillaries. Weather affects skin in several ways; cold winds, strong sunlight and extremes of temperature all encourage the development of telangiectasia, especially where the surface capillary network is weak.

## Contra-indications to treatment

- *AIDS:* acquired-immune deficiency syndrome caused by the human immune deficiency virus, which is easily transmitted via the bloodstream. Treatment of telangiectasia involves inserting a sterile needle into the blood supply. Therefore treatment carries a slight risk of cross-infection. According to Dr Noah, *Hygienic Skin Piercing 1988,* evidence has shown that HIV which causes AIDS is less infectious and more sensitive than the hepatitis B virus. HIV has been shown to be more sensitive and therefore inactivated after a short period of time in the environment.
- *Allergies:* With allergic tendencies the skin flushes easily. Recurrent erythema puts stress on weakened capillary structures. Treatment will not be successful unless the main irritant is avoided.
- *Asthma:* See contra-indication to electrical epilation, page 134. Due to the impaired oxygen supply to the skin the healing process is slower. The problem will recur in a very short period of time due to the capillary network being weaker.
- *Drugs:* such as anti-coagulants, e.g. warfarin prevent clotting of the blood. Clients requiring anti-coagulant drugs usually have a problem with the cardio-vascular system.
- *Dermographic skins:* show an adverse reaction to the needle. Wheals and/or oedema occur where the needle has entered the skin. The healing rate is slower, with the skin taking some time to return to normal.
- *Diabetes:* the skin is slower to heal, with the client's pain threshold being considerably lower.
- *Epilepsy:* due to the precision work relating to the removal of telangiectasia, treatment is best avoided. This is because stress of the application of a high-frequency current could interfere with the electrical impulses of the brain. A fit could be brought on in this way. Should treatment be given, the doctor's authorization must be obtained prior to commencement.
- *Haemophilia:* is contra-indicated to this treatment due to the malfunction of the clotting mechanism.
- *Hay fever:* results in frequent sneezing which in turn can rupture the superficial capillaries, particularly around the nose.
- *Hepatitis B:* is highly infectious and the virus is not destroyed easily. Spider naevi occur in large numbers. Once the condition has been cleared, which takes some considerable time, spider naevi may be

treated. However the client must consult their doctor and obtain the doctor's written agreement.

- *Hepatitis C.*
- *Hypertension:* Nerve endings are highly sensitive. Due to the client's inability to relax there is a risk of scarring if the client pulls away while the current is flowing.
- *Keloid scarring:* is an over-growth of skin tissue at the site of an injury. There is a slight possibility that keloids could develop where the needle has entered the skin.
- *Pregnancy:* naevi which appear during pregnancy often disappear within a few months after the birth. Therefore these are best left untreated.
- *Rosacea:* although this condition cannot be cleared completely by short-wave diathermy the appearance can be improved considerably. Liaison with the client's doctor is advisable prior to treatment.
- *Vascular disorders:* result in a weakened surface capillary network. Treatment is unlikely to be successful.

## Consultation procedure

As with electrical epilation a full case history should be taken prior to treatment. The procedure is similar. Full medical history and details of medications should be noted. Any history of serious illness requires a doctor's letter prior to treatment. For the benefit of both the client and the therapist it is advisable to treat a small test patch. This will enable the therapist to observe the skin's reaction and will let the client know how the treatment feels.

In addition the consultation should include discussion of the following: the type of skin (sensitivity, healing rate, tendency to bruise); nature of employment, (e.g. hot, steamy kitchens, outdoors); diet (tea/coffee/alcohol intake, hot spicy foods); smoking; frequency and temperature of baths; circulatory disorders (heart problems); asthma; hay fever; sinus problems; operations (blood transfusions); hepatitis B and disorders associated with the liver.

Contra-indications for electrical epilation also apply for advanced epilation techniques.

## Equipment and materials needed for treatment

- Shortwave diathermy machine or blend unit
- Magnifying lamp
- Sterilized disposable needles
- Sharps box for contaminated needles
- Sterile forceps for removal of needles from chuck after treatment
- Antiseptic solution
- Cotton wool
- Aftercare lotion
- Camera (optional extra which can be most useful, particularly when treatment takes place over a long period of time)

## Method of treatment for telangiectasia by shortwave diathermy

1 Check the condition of the skin. Refer to the consultation/record card.
2 Remove any traces of make-up in the area. Cleanse the skin thoroughly and wipe over with mild antiseptic solution such as Hibitaine. Examine the results of the patch test.
3 Insert pre-sterilized disposable needle into the chuck.
4 Find the feeder vein. Hold the skin taut with the fingers of both hands.

139

Gently stroke to drain the vein. Look carefully to find the direction from which the vein is filling.

5 Apply the needle lightly to the end of the capillary. Leave sufficient healing gaps. Coagulation takes places on a very low setting. Care must be taken not to burn the skin's surface. Application time should be kept to a minimum. For effective results it is essential that the skin is not over-treated.

6 Treat larger veins first.

7 On completion of treatment aftercare lotion such as lacto-calamine, Witch Doctor or similar should be applied.

Precise instructions on homecare routine should be given at this stage. The importance of this must be stressed to the client.

8 Allow a minimum of three to four weeks before giving further treatment in the same area.

## Skin's response to treatment

1 Blanching of the skin on application of current.
2 Erythema.
3 Oedema – raised lumps, which is a reaction to the needle.
4 Scabs may appear after two to three days. These must not be scratched or picked off, but allowed to fall off naturally in their own time.
5 When treating naevi they may appear to look worse for up to two weeks.
6 Leg veins take up to three or four weeks to heal. Treatment of small veins on the legs is not to be recommended by shortwave diathermy. Due to a number of factors such as pressure on the main veins and the depth of the feeder veins the problem often recurs within a short period of time.

The use of an SLR camera with a close-up lens can be a definite advantage. Photographs should be taken at the beginning of treatment, in the middle of the course, and at the conclusion. Where treatment sessions span a period of time, the client can often forget the extent of the initial problem. The production of before and after photographs is encouraging for the client and provides a visual record for the therapist.

## Treatment of spider naevi and Campbell de Morgan spots

Both spider naevi and Campbell de Morgan spots can be removed easily with shortwave diathermy or blend. Before treating either, any make up in the area should be removed and the skin wiped with antiseptic solution.

*Spider naevi* are best treated by inserting a sterile needle into the main body of the naevi and applying the current. The shortwave diathermy coagulates the feeder capillary, so depriving the rest of the naevus of its blood supply. A scab can sometimes form at the point of needle insertion. Clients should be advised to allow any scab to fall off naturally and that it should not be picked off. A scab is less likely to form when blend is used for treatment.

*Campbell de Morgan* spots respond well to treatment by shortwave diathermy and blend. A sterile needle is inserted into the side of the spot and the current applied. The current intensity should be sufficiently high to coagulate, yet not so high that skin damage occurs.

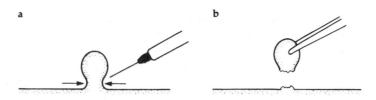

**Figure 17.1** Removal of a skin tag

**a** Apply heat to neck of tag at junction with epidermis
**b** Lift treated tag with sterile forceps

# Treatment of skin tags

## Equipment

- Sterile needles, sizes 5, 6 or 10
- Sterile forceps/tweezers
- Shortwave diathermy or blend machine
- Antiseptic solution
- Sterile dressings, for areas where friction may occur, e.g. underarm, waist, etc.

## Procedure using shortwave diathermy

1 Swab area with antiseptic solution.
2 Select and insert sterile needle.
3 Turn up the current to a high intensity.
4 While holding the skin tag with sterile forceps apply the current to the neck of the tag at the junction with the skin's surface.
5 When the skin tag has been removed apply aftercare and a sterile dressing where necessary.

## Procedure using Blend technique

1 Swab area with antiseptic solution.
2 Select and insert sterile needle.
3 Turn galvanic and high frequency currents to required intensity.
4 While holding the skin tag with sterile forceps apply the current to the neck of the tag at the junction of the skin's surface. The tag will not dry out as with shortwave diathermy but will begin to liquefy at the junction of the skin. The skin heals faster.

The removal of skin tags, moles or warts *should not* be undertaken by any therapist without the necessary training with a reputable instructor. Due to the specialist nature of this work full instructions for treatment are not given in this text. These must be obtained during training. When considering training it is advisable to contact the specialist professional associations for their list of recognized tutors.

For insurance purposes it is necessary to obtain a *written* note from the client's doctor before the commencement of treatment.

**Qualifying criteria for acceptance on to Advanced Epilation Courses CIBTAC:**
Two thousand hours documented post qualifying experience or 5 years continuous practice in electrical epilation.

**Qualifying criteria for BAE members wishing to sit for the advanced epilation examination:**
Five years post qualifying experience in practical electrical epilation.

**Qualifying criteria for Institute of Electrolysis members:**
Five years post qualifying experience in practical electrical epilation.

**Review questions**

1 Define the term 'telangiectasia'.
2 Name and explain the conditions which either cause or aggravate telangiectasia.
3 Explain why the following are contra-indications to treatment:
   (a) asthma;
   (b) haemophilia;
   (c) hay fever;
   (d) keloid scarring.
4 State the additional information required during an initial consultation for advanced electrical epilation treatment.
5 Describe the application of treatment for telangiectasia.
6 Describe the procedure for the removal of skin tags.

# 18 Hygiene and sterilization

The importance of attention to detail with regard to staff hygiene, cleaning and sterilization practises in the clinic cannot be over-stressed. During the late 1980s mass media attention on the subject of AIDS gave rise to uneasiness and fear of the unknown among the general public and in turn led to clients becoming more aware of the risk of infection from the use of contaminated needles.

The electrolysist should take measures to prevent all cross-infection. Viruses that cause particular concern among clients are HIV, hepatitis B and C, which are transmitted by blood and blood-stained body fluids. Cases of infection through blood infected with HIV and hepatitis, by surgery, blood transfusion, acupuncture and dental treatment, have been recorded.

The main aim is to avoid cross-infection from one client to another, and from the client to the electrolysist or vice versa. This can be achieved easily by:

1   Carrying out thorough cleaning of treatment rooms
2   Cleaning and sterilization of all equipment, forceps and needles.
3   Attention to personal hygiene.
4   Keeping cuts and abrasions covered.
5   Handwashing after all client contact.
6   Correct disposal of clinic waste.

Provided that every care is taken, the risk of cross-infection during electro-epilation is minimal.

There are a number of terms with which the practising electrolysist should be familiar:

* *Bacteria:* small one-cell micro-organisms which need a moist warm atmosphere in order to survive. They also need oxygen, and they give out carbon dioxide. Some bacteria are harmless to the human body, for example, those found in the digestive tract. Others are responsible for conditions such as impetigo, food poisoning and boils.
* *Bactericide:* a chemical agent which will kill most bacteria but which is not effective on viruses.
* *Virus:* minute particles which are completely inactive outside the living cells they infect. In suitable environments they are capable of reproduction and mutation (W. G. Peberdy, *Sterilisation and Hygiene*, 1988). Examples of viral infections are influenza, the common cold, hepatitis A, B, C and D and HIV.
* *Asepsis:* the absence of infection from micro-organisms.

- *Aseptic:* free from organisms capable of causing disease.
- *Sepsis:* presence of infection due to micro-organisms.
- *Sterilization:* the process used to achieve total destruction of all living organisms and spores.

## HIV/AIDS

The full name for AIDS is acquired immune deficiency syndrome, which develops as a result of infection by the human immuno-deficiency virus (HIV).

The virus can be transmitted by infected blood entering the body through heterosexual or homosexual contact, entry into open wounds, contaminated hypodermic, acupuncture or electro-epilation needles.

Cases of infection after a small percentage of blood transfusions from an infected donor in the 1980s have been recorded.

HIV-positive means the virus is present in the body and over a period of time will impair the body's defence mechanism by interfering with the immune system, which has developed from the HIV.

HIV interferes with the immune system so reducing the body's ability to cope effectively with disease or infection such as pneumonia. It is these secondary infections which often prove fatal. A person who is HIV positive may show any or all of the following symptoms:

1 General fatigue.
2 Inability to recover fully from infections such as colds or influenza.
3 Enlargement of the lymph nodes.
4 Weight loss.
5 Diarrhoea.

The HIV is a fragile virus when exposed to air, and is one that is easily destroyed by the use of disinfectants.

## Hepatitis

The hepatitis A, B, C, D and E viruses are far more resilient than HIV and are capable of existing for considerable periods of time on infected needles and hard surfaces.

The name 'hepatitis' means 'inflammation of the liver'. There are four categories of virus causing hepatitis:

1 *Hepatitis type A,* infective hepatitis, also known as short incubation hepatitis. Causes diarrhoea and vomiting. It is spread by the faecal, oral route.
2 *Hepatitis type B-serum,* also known as long incubation hepatitis, affects the liver and is transmitted by blood.
3 *HCV,* formerly known as non-A and non-B hepatitis.
4 *HDV and HEV,* as yet there is very little documented information on these specific viruses.

*Hepatitis A* is of short duration, with an incubation period of approximately one month. This particular virus can be contracted from contaminated food or water. The hepatitis A virus is lost from the body fairly quickly.

*Hepatitis B* is a far more serious condition of longer duration. The incubation period varies from between 40 to 150 days, during which time the patient is highly infectious.

The person infected with hepatitis B feels generally unwell and fatigued for a lengthy period of time, e.g. several months. This is followed by a long convalescence. Symptoms shown in the early stages include nausea, vomiting, loss of appetite and general fatigue. The whites of the eyes, together with the skin and gums, may take on a yellow appearance. Fever may also be present in the early stages of infection. Unlike hepatitis A, the B virus remains in the body for a considerable length of time.

The hepatitis B virus may readily be transmitted by contaminated needles and blood. It has been found that the virus can remain inactive on hard surfaces for several years, therefore high standards of hygiene in the clinic are imperative.

Vaccination against hepatitis B is possible and indeed advisable for people working in high-risk occupations. Procedure consists of three vaccinations, the first two at an interval of one month with the third at six months. Details and information can be obtained from a doctor's surgery.

*Hepatitis C* is blood-borne and lies between A and B in severity. Symptoms which are similar to those of flu are gradual in their onset and are milder than those of hepatitis A and B. The incubation period is between 20 days and thirteen weeks. There is no vaccine available for hepatitis C. Acquisition is through the use of infected syringes in drug users, where syringes are used by more than one person, post blood transfusion and occupational exposure.

## Clinic hygiene

Hygiene within the clinic is easily achieved and the procedure should be a routine matter. All equipment, hard work surfaces and washable floors should be wiped over daily with a hospital grade disinfectant. There are many of these available on the market, a number of which are environmentally friendly. Hand wash basins should be cleaned regularly. Soap bars should be placed in a soap rack between use. Soap pump dispensers are more hygienic. Hands should be dried on disposable paper towels.

When using disinfectants for the purpose of killing viruses and bacterial spores it is essential that the manufacturer's instructions for dilution percentage are strictly adhered to. Accurate timing for immersion of objects in disinfectant is important.

The disadvantage of some of the strong disinfectants is the risk of skin irritation or allergies. A few may not be environmentally friendly, which causes problems when disposing of the solution.

Solutions containing chlorhexidine have a high level of antibacterial activity with low toxicity which should be used after washing with soap to disinfect the hands prior to giving treatment and preparing the skin for electro-epilation.

Once made into solution, a majority of disinfectant and antiseptic preparations have a limited shelf life and it is wise, therefore, to be guided by the manufacturer's recommendations.

Treatment couches should be covered with fresh disposable paper towels for each client. Used clinic waste, such as paper towels, cotton wool swabs, tissues and disposable gloves, should be placed in a covered container lined with a plastic bag. The plastic bag should be securely tied and disposed of daily.

Surfaces contaminated by blood should be cleaned using disposable gloves and paper towels, which should then be discarded into a plastic bag.

Containers holding contaminated probes/forceps should be cleaned and sterilized daily. Instruments which have been dropped on the floor should be washed and re-sterilized prior to use.

## Needles

Although it is possible to sterilize needles with an autoclave, the use of pre-sterilized disposable needles rules out the possibility of cross-infection from one client to another particularly as far as HIV or hepatitis are concerned.

Disposable needles are sterilized in one of two ways:

1 Needles packed in hospital-grade blister packs sterilized with ethylene oxide gas.
2 Individually packed needles sterilized by gamma irradiation – these packets have a red dot on the outside which proves that sterilization has taken place.

After use needles should be placed in a sharps box.

When sterilizing needles by other methods the following procedures should be adhered to. Mechanically pre-clean the needles by using swabs or cotton balls moistened with a solution of low residue detergent or a protein dissolving enzyme detergent and cool water.

Needles should then be submerged in a holding container filled with a solution of low residue detergent or a protein dissolving enzyme, then rinsed and dried.

After cleaning, needles and instruments should be sterilized by placing in a dry heat oven or an autoclave.

### Sterilization methods
*Dry heat*

180°C (350°F) for 30 minutes
170°C (340°F) for one hour
160°C (320°F) for two hours

*Moist heat (steam under pressure) – autoclave*

Time of exposure should follow the manufacturer's recommended guide-line:

1 15 minutes at 121°C (250°F) 15 psi (pounds per square inch) for unpackaged instruments/items.
2 30 minutes at 121°C (250°F) 15 psi for packaged instruments/items.

The above times are for exposure once the specified temperature has been reached. This does not include heating up time.

## Needle stick injury

To prevent needle stick injury, disposable and damaged/bent needles should not be straightened or otherwise manipulated by hand, but placed in a puncture-resistant container (sharps box) which is securely sealed. The sharps box should be disposed of in the manner specified by the local health regulations or, in the USA, by the State.

*Note:* In the USA the FDA have not as yet approved the use of glass-bead sterilizers. It would appear that glass-bead sterilizers do not comply with the recommendations made by the Medical Devices Agency of the Department of Health (UK) for methods of sterilization (January 1995)

**Figure 18.1** Inserting sterile two-piece needle into needle holder

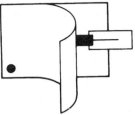

**a** Loosen cap of needle holder, ready to insert needle
**b** Peel open sealed packet; remove sterile needle with sterile forceps

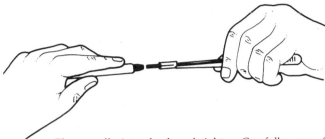

**c** Place needle into chuck and tighten. Carefully ease off protective cap by gently twisting and pulling

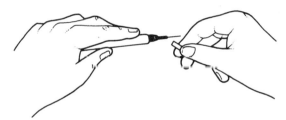

**d** Adjust needle by loosening cap of needle holder, using end of protective cover

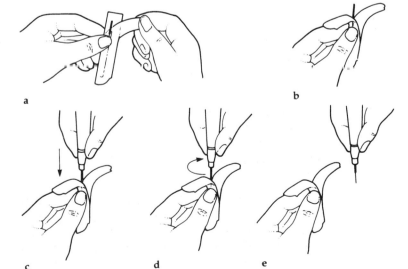

a

b

**Figure 18.2** Inserting sterile one-piece needle into needle holder

c

d

e

## Needle holders, caps, chucks and forceps

Needle holders should be wiped over with a detergent solution – germicide/disinfectant after each treatment. Plastic or metal caps, chucks and forceps should be immersed in a disinfectant solution for at least one hour, then rinsed in water and dried with tissue or paper towel prior to use, or cleaned with soap/detergent and water, rinsed then immersed in 70% isopropyl alcohol for at least ten minutes. The covered container used to hold the alcohol should be emptied daily or whenever visibly contaminated.

Forceps, metal caps and chucks are all suitable for sterilization in an autoclave.

The advent of the Ballet ejector needle holder, developed by Arand Ltd, is an innovation in the field of electro-epilation. This needle holder contains an internal spring activated mechanism, which allows the epilation needle to be inserted and removed from the needle holder automatically when the electrolysist presses the ejector button. There is no need for the operator to touch the needle with either forceps or fingers. The risk of needle stick injury to the electrolosist is reduced due to the needles being ejected directly into the sharps box.

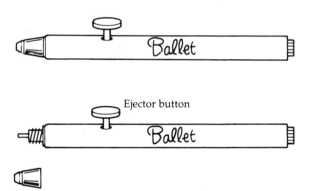

**Figure 18.3** Ballet ejector needle holder

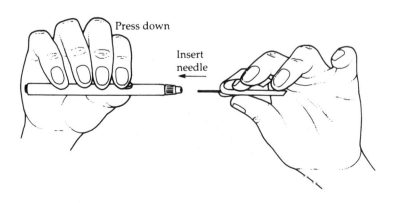

**Figure 18.4** Loading ejector needle

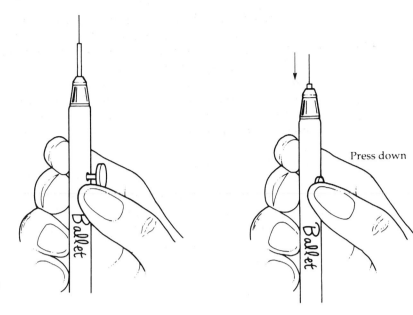

**Figure 18.5** Setting the needle

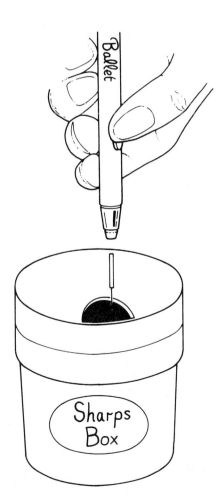

**Figure 18.6** Disposing of used needle

## Disposable materials

Consumables such as cotton wool pads and tissues, which may be used to protect the client's eyes against the light, and disposable gloves should be used once only and then discarded into a lined, covered container. The treatment couch or plinth should be covered with fresh disposable paper towels for each client. Bin liners should be replaced daily. Sharps boxes containing contaminated needles and micro-lances should be collected by the local Department of the Environment on request or, arrangements should be made with the local hospital.

## Hand preparation prior to treatment

The hands should be washed, preferably with liquid soap or bactericidal preparations immediately before and after treatment.

All cuts, abrasions or open wounds should be covered with a waterproof dressing prior to treatment. When a number of cuts or open wounds are present the use of disposable gloves is essential.

The use of a fresh pair of disposable surgical gloves is recommended for each client. These should be changed when damaged or after any interruption to treatments.

## Preparation of area to be treated

All make-up in the area should be removed. Chlorhexidine solution or a spirit swab may be used to wipe the area prior to treatment, and the cotton wool or swab should be discarded immediately. Skin should then be dried with a disposable tissue prior to probing. Surgical spirit is not recommended due to its flammable properties and its drying effect on the skin.

## Sterilization methods

Sterilization is achieved in a number of ways:

1 Disposable needles by ethylene oxide gas or gamma irradiation.
2 Metal instruments such as scissors, forceps, metal caps and removable chucks by autoclave.
3 Chemical disinfectants (not recommended for needles or forceps used for treatment).

### Autoclaves

An autoclave is a piece of equipment which allows certain items such as needles, forceps and scissors to be sterilized by steam at temperatures of 121°C under pressure. Modern autoclaves have thermochromic indicators which change colour when the required temperature has been reached. A stacking system is usually provided so that the items can be placed at different levels in the autoclave. Temperatures range from 121°C to 134°C and with correct time and heat exposure kill all spores. However some materials can be unfavourably affected by the temperature range.

*Note:* Information relating to standards of sterilization of electrolysis implements recommended by the Centres for Disease Control was supplied by James Paisner, Synoptic Products, USA; and John Fantz RE, former State Examiner, USA.

### Activated glutaraldehyde solutions

Glutaraldehyde is effective in destroying vegetative bacteria, spores and fungi. The effective life span of activated glutaraldehyde varies from 14 to 28 days, and therefore manufacturers' recommendations should be followed.

**Figure 18.7** An
autoclave

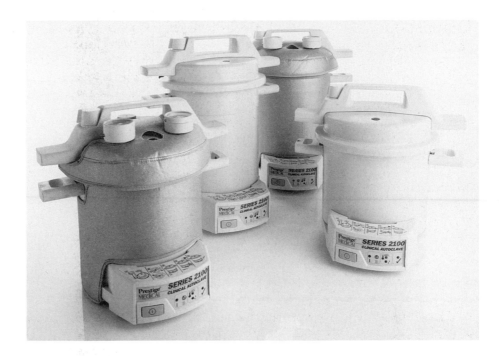

## Personal hygiene

The electrolysist's general appearance and personal hygiene give an insight into the character of the individual. Untidy hair, bad breath, soiled overalls, scuffed shoes and grubby fingernails give a slipshod impression. On the other hand, well-groomed hair, short manicured nails, clean shoes, a newly laundered uniform and fresh breath all contribute to a smart, well cared for appearance which will not be missed by the clients.

A daily bath or shower and regular use of deodorant should be routine. Clinic uniform benefits from being changed daily. For those electrolysists who must smoke, care should be taken to ensure that tobacco odour does not cling to the breath, hair, skin, hands or uniform. Stale tobacco can be most offensive to the non-smoking client or colleague. Smoking should be confined to social hours only.

Strong foods such as curry, garlic or onions are inclined to cling to the breath and should therefore be avoided prior to and during clinic hours. Teeth should be brushed regularly.

## Local Government (Miscellaneous Provisions) Act 1982: Health and Safety at Work Act 1974

These Acts give the local health inspector from the Department of the Environment power to enter and inspect the premises without notice. The local authority also has the power to close down any business which does not comply with the regulations laid down in the Acts relating to standards of safety, health and hygiene. Details relating to both these Acts can be found in Chapter 20.

**Review questions**

1 Define the following terms:
   (a) asepsis
   (b) antiseptic
   (c) disinfectant
   (d) sterilization
   (e) bactericide.
2 State the difference between a disinfectant and an antiseptic.
3 State the aim of hygiene and sterilization procedures in the clinic.
4 (a) Describe the following: 'bacteria'; 'virus'.
   (b) Name two infections caused by each of these.
5 What do the initials HIV stand for?
6 How does HIV affect the human body?
7 What do the initials AIDS stand for?
8 List the symptoms which may be present when a person is HIV positive.
9 Explain the difference between HIV and AIDS.
10 State the incubation periods for:
   (a) hepatitis A
   (b) hepatitis B
   (c) hepatitis C.
11 Explain the ways in which HIV and hepatitis B can be transmitted.
12 List the symptoms associated with hepatitis B.
13 Name two methods for sterilizing disposable needles.
14 Describe ways in which forceps may be sterilized.
15 Give the reason for covering cuts and abrasions on hands prior to giving treatment.
16 List and describe four methods of sterilization.

# 19 First aid

It is advisable for each member of staff to undergo first-aid training to the standards laid down by the St John Ambulance Brigade, The British Red Cross Association or the St Andrew's Ambulance Association (Scotland). Certificates are valid for three years, after which time a refresher course and re-examination are recommended.

The first-aid manual authorized by all three associations stresses that life-saving techniques of artificial ventilation and external chest compression should not be given by a person who has not been trained in the techniques.

When giving first-aid treatment the following points should be observed:

1  the situation should be assessed without endangering either the life of the casualty or the person giving the first aid;
2  identify the condition from which the casualty is suffering;
3  administer the relevant first-aid treatment;
4  where necessary summon a doctor or emergency services;
5  after the casualty has been attended to enter all details relating to the incident in a report book.

The aim of this chapter is to cover the situations that are most likely to occur in the clinic. Full details of all emergency and first aid procedures are covered in the *First-aid Manual* of the St John Ambulance Brigade, The British Red Cross Society and the St Andrew's Association, 5th edition, 1987.

## First aid box

In order to meet the requirements of the Health and Safety at Work Act 1981 every clinic should have a first aid box which contains the following:

1  a selection of individually wrapped sterile adhesive dressings;
2  sterile bandages, including triangular bandages;
3  sterile eye pad;
4  sterilized non-medicated dressings;
5  safety pins;
6  a record book for recording details of all incidents requiring first aid attention;
7  cotton wool, tweezers and a pair of scissors.

The first-aid box should be kept in a visible and easily accessible position.

## The recovery position

The recovery position (see Figure 19.1) is used when a casualty is breathing, has a heartbeat, but is unconscious. The purpose of this position is to prevent the casualty's tongue falling to the back of the throat, and to keep the air passages open and free from obstructions.

1  Turn the casualty on to one side, ensuring that the head is supported.
2  Place the arm at right angles to the upper body, with the elbow bent.

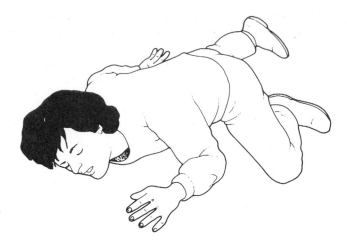

**Figure 19.1** The recovery position

3 Bend the upper leg, and place at right angles to the body.
4 With the casualty's head turned to one side, tilt the head back with the jaw forward to ensure an open airway is maintained.

## Burns and scalds

The type of burn will depend on the cause of injury. The nature and size of the burn will determine the treatment to be given. Severe burns or burns covering a large area may give rise to shock, and hospital treatment may be necessary.

- *Dry burns* are caused by fire, lighted cigarettes, electrical equipment or friction.
- *Scalds* are caused by wet heat such as a boiling kettle, very hot liquids such as water, tea or coffee and hot oil or fat.
- *Cold burns* may be caused by contact with freezing cold metals.
- *Chemical burns* may be caused by the skin coming into contact with alkaline or acid substances. Mild chemical burns to the skin may occur if the indifferent electrode held by the client during galvanic electrolysis is not covered in damp viscose, cotton wool or similar. However this is easily prevented when the treatment procedure is carried out correctly.
- *Electrical burns* can easily be the result of too much heat produced by an electrical current, e.g. high frequency. This can occur when the high-frequency intensity during shortwave diathermy is too high and the underlying skin tissue or surface is burnt. Electrical burns can also be caused by lightning.
- *Radiation burns* can occur as a result of over-exposure to sunlight or snow. Rays from the sun reflect off the snow and in severe cases can cause long-term damage to either skin or eyes.
- *Blisters* appear on the surface where the skin has been damaged by either friction or heat. They are raised swellings which contain tissue fluid. Blisters should not be broken as there is a risk of infection occurring. In time the blister will dry up without assistance.

**General treatment of burns**

The aim is to reduce heat and pain in the area, prevent infection and lessen the effects of shock. Medical attention or hospitalization may be necessary in severe cases.

When possible, place the affected area under cold running water for a minimum of 10 minutes. For areas that cannot be placed under running water, bathe well with cold water. Restrictive clothing, belts or jewellery should be removed before any swelling appears, but do not try to remove anything that has become stuck to the burn. Once the pain and heat have been reduced cover the area with dry, sterile dressing. Ointments, lotions and fats such as butter *should not* be applied to the burn.

# Choking

This occurs when the air passages have become totally or partly blocked by an obstruction. This may be the result of food or drink going down the wrong way, and sometimes through an obstruction in the throat. The aim is to remove the obstruction and restore breathing to normal as quickly as possible.

Encourage the casualty to cough. If this fails to dislodge the obstruction, remove any false teeth from the mouth and ask the casualty to lean forward with the head in a lower position than the lungs. Apply short, sharp slaps between the shoulder blades with the heel of the hand.

# Concussion

This occurs as a result of a fall, or a blow to the head or jaw which may or may not result in loss of consciousness. The casualty may be confused and unable to remember events immediately prior to or after the incident. A careful eye should be kept on the casualty when there is a possibility that concussion has occurred, and should there be any deterioration in the condition, or should symptoms persist, the casualty must be referred for medical attention urgently.

If necessary carry out the procedure for loss of consciousness. On recovery from concussion check the pulse rate and breathing. Treat for shock if applicable. Do not give liquids to drink in case the casualty needs to be removed to hospital. Head injuries can be serious and may result in long-term damage.

# Diabetes

A diabetic needs to maintain a careful balance of the blood-sugar level. This is usually achieved by the use of either insulin injections or tablets. If insufficient food is eaten, a prolonged period elapses between meals, or too much insulin is taken, the concentration of sugar in the blood will drop. This can affect the brain and could result in unconsciousness or even death.

When the blood-sugar level drops, the diabetic person may feel faint and light-headed, confused and may appear drunk. Other signs are pale skin, with profuse sweating, rapid pulse rate, shallow breathing and shaking limbs.

First-aid treatment is to restore the blood sugar level as quickly as possible. This can be achieved by giving the conscious casualty sweet liquids to drink or sugar-lumps to eat. If the casualty responds, give further sweetened food or liquid within a few minutes. On recovery the diabetic should seek medical advice. When consciousness is lost the ambulance should be called immediately and the casualty transferred to hospital.

## Epileptic fits

These occur when there is a temporary disruption to the normal electrical activity of the brain. Fits may be minor or major and may last from a few seconds to several minutes.

Symptoms which occur immediately before and during an epileptic fit are inattentiveness, licking of the lips, incoherence and possibly loss of memory. During the fit the casualty may fall to the floor and lose consciousness.

The casualty may become rigid for a few seconds, and sometimes loses bladder control. After the fit is over the casualty may be a little confused and will be in need of reassurance.

The aim of first aid during an epileptic fit is to protect the casualty from injury. Clear a space in the surrounding area by moving any equipment, furniture or obstacles out of the way. Should the casualty fall, loosen clothing around the neck and place a soft pillow or some form of support under the head. *Do not* try to restrain or lift the casualty in any way and *do not* put anything into the mouth. After the fit, reassurance should be given but drinks are not advisable until the casualty is fully alert. It will not be necessary to call an ambulance unless an injury has occurred, the casualty has taken longer than fifteen minutes to regain consciousness, or has several fits in quick succession.

## Fainting

This can be described as a temporary loss of consciousness brought about by the reduction of blood supply to the brain. There are a number of reasons why this may occur: lack of fresh air, as in a hot, stuffy room; lack of food; emotional shock; physical exhaustion.

The casualty may become pale and dizzy or feel unsteady. The aim of first aid treatment is to encourage the flow of blood to the brain. When the casualty feels faint, place her in a sitting position, leaning forward with the head between the knees. Encourage deep breathing. Alternatively when the casualty has fainted lie her down, raise the legs and loosen restrictive clothing around the waist and chest. Ensure that there is sufficient fresh air in the area.

## Heat exhaustion and heat stroke

These are conditions which arise through the body becoming overheated. Body salts and water are lost in both instances.

Heat exhaustion usually occurs after physical exercise in hot, moist conditions. Heat stroke occurs after exposure to heat or high humidity.

Symptoms of heat exhaustion are headaches, nausea and dizziness. Muscular cramps may also occur due to salt loss. The casualty's skin may become pale, breathing may be shallow, pulse rate weak and the casualty may faint. The aim is to restore lost body fluids as soon as possible by giving sips of cold water. When cramps are present half a teaspoon of salt should be added to half a litre of water. The casualty should be moved to a cool place and medical aid called if necessary.

Symptoms of heat stroke are a little different, usually dizziness, nausea, headache and increased body temperature. In severe cases the casualty may lose consciousness. The aim of first aid is to reduce the body temperature as quickly as possible. This may be achieved by moving the casualty to a cool area, using an electric fan to encourage the circulation of air in the immediate area, placing the casualty in a direct current of air or covering with a cold wet sheet. A doctor should be contacted.

## Insect stings

Bees and wasps cause stings which are more painful and alarming than they are dangerous. There are some people, however who have an allergic reaction to the poison. Stings in the mouth and throat may cause swelling, leading to asphyxia.

Signs and symptoms may be unexpected sharp pain, swelling around the affected area. Shock may occur depending on the degree of reaction.

The sting should be removed with forceps. Pain and swelling should be relieved by the application of a cold compress, surgical spirit or a solution of bicarbonate of soda.

When the sting is in the mouth give the casualty ice to suck in order to reduce the swelling, or rinse the mouth with a solution of bicarbonate of soda and water, or cold water. If the casualty experiences breathing difficulties place in the recovery position.

## Shock

This may occur as a result of any one of the following:

1 distressing news such as the death of a close relative or friend;
2 an accident;
3 the witnessing of an unpleasant situation such as a road traffic accident;
4 injury to the body, e.g. electrical shock, burns or severe bleeding.

General circulation is affected, with the body directing the available blood to the vital organs, e.g. brain, heart and kidneys, leaving insufficient oxygen and blood available for the remaining organs to function efficiently. Severe shock can result in death.

Signs of shock are as follows:

1 the skin becomes pale, cold and moist;
2 pulse rate is weak;
3 nausea and dizziness may be present;
4 loss of consciousness in some instances.

Medical help should be called and severe cases removed to hospital. The casualty should be reassured until medical help arrives, but under no circumstances should food or drink be given which would delay the administration of anaesthetic should it be necessary.

## Summoning the emergency services in the UK

In an emergency situation both time and lives may be saved when the emergency services are called quickly and efficiently. The procedure is very simple.

1 Using the nearest telephone dial 999.
2 Name the emergency service required, i.e. ambulance, police, fire.
3 Give the telephone number from which you are calling, together with the exact location of the emergency.
4 State the nature of the emergency and the number of casualties involved.
5 Ensure information given is both clear and concise.
6 Return to the location of the incident and await the arrival of the relevant service.

**Report book**

It is advisable to keep a record book in the clinic. This should be used to record accurate details of any incident or accident that occurs on the premises.

The details that should be entered are the date, time and location of the incident, the name and address of the person involved, the nature of the incident, any first aid given and action taken. There is always the possibility that this information may be needed at a later date either for the casualty's doctor, or in the event of a possible lawsuit.

**Review questions**

1   Explain the purpose of first aid.
2   List the items that should be available in the first aid box.
3   Where should the first aid box be kept?
4   (a)  Describe the recovery position.
     (b)  Explain the purpose of the recovery position.
5   Describe the first aid treatment for:
     (a) a chemical burn
     (b) an electrical burn.
6   Explain why blisters should not be broken.
7   State the first aid procedure for concussion.
8   What is the aim of first aid in relation to an epileptic fit?
9   Give the signs and symptoms of an impending faint.
10   (a)  Explain the difference between heat exhaustion and heat stroke.
     (b)  Describe the first aid treatment for both the above conditions.
11   List the signs and symptoms of shock.
12   Describe the procedure for summoning the emergency services in the UK.
13   What is the purpose of the report book?

# 20 Starting and running a business

The ambition of many students at the start of training is eventually to have their own business. It is a sad fact that a high percentage of business ventures fail in the first three years. This is due to a number of reasons, however with careful planning and preparation in advance many of the risks of failure can be minimized.

Many decide to go it alone to escape the constrictions of being an employee, or because of the shortage of good employers and jobs available. The more positive reasons are job satisfaction, financial rewards and independence. Those looking for shorter hours and longer holidays will be disappointed.

Commitment is essential. Those who research the idea thoroughly, look into all the potential problems, and produce a sound business plan are more likely to succeed.

Due to the vast volume of information relating to business studies, it is not possible to deal with the subject matter in any great depth in this book. The aim of this section is to give an insight into the planning, setting up and running of a small business.

**Initial steps to success**

1 Remember that the key figure who determines success is the owner or proprietor. Setting up in business means being the driving force and having total commitment, self-discipline and determination.

2 Market research is essential in order to assess how many people are likely to require the services on offer; how many competitors are established in the area; the prices being charged by competitors.

3 Creating the right image for the business is important. The name chosen should convey a professional image and get the message across. It is advisable to check that no other business has the same name.

4 People who make a detailed business plan are more likely to succeed. This is one of the keys to success, and it should include realistic trading and cashflow projections. Without this plan, finance will be hard to raise. The best plans are often those drawn up with professional help.

5 Finance and funding are two major hurdles. A well-prepared and thought out business plan is a valuable asset when raising finance. Your own bank is probably the first place to approach and it may well be able to provide all or part of the finance required. Business premises and equipment are best financed by medium to long-term loans, whereas day-to-day working capital requirements are usually provided by a fluctuating overdraft facility. There is also a wide range

6 The services of a good, professionally qualified accountant, bank manager and solicitor are essential. The services of a reputable insurance broker are also an asset. Each provides a valuable service, and the safest method of finding these professionals is by personal recommendation. The accountant will advise on finances, cashflow, VAT registration and returns, and Inland Revenue requirements. Other areas that will need to be looked at, are the arranging of insurance and the drawing up of legal business documents. Legal and leasing agreements should be checked by experts. Every step should be taken to ensure that legal requirements are met.

7 The location of the business is important. Thought needs to be given to the surrounding location, ease of access, parking, public transport and number of potential clients in the area. Competition in the immediate area should also be considered. Research into any future development plans projected for nearby and surrounding areas should be undertaken.

8 Equipment should be looked at. Requirements, availability, and delivery dates should be researched, as should the manner by which the equipment is to be paid for – cash, hire purchase or leasing.

9 When there is a possibility that the first year's turnover will exceed the VAT registration level it is advisable to register with the Customs and Excise at the start of trading.

10 A simple accounts procedure should be set up.

11 The Inland Revenue must be informed of the proposed business. When employing staff, ensure that the employment laws are met and contracts drawn up.

## Business plan

When starting a business, particularly when funding is required, a well-researched and prepared business plan goes a long way to getting the business started, and raising necessary finance. The plan should be well-prepared, typed neatly and presented in a folder.

The business plan should include:

1 Name and address of the business.
2 Name of the company or person who has prepared the plan.
3 Position of the above in the proposed business, for example proprietor.
4 Purpose and main activity of the business, for example electrolysis.
5 Premises – location, ease of access, public transport, parking facilities. State how the premises would be set up, for example number of treatment rooms, reception, stock room, staff room.
6 Benefits of the proposed business to the proprietor or partners.
7 Competition – their strengths and weaknesses.
8 Capital costs.
9 Running costs.
10 Income – sources, for example treatments, retail sales, etc.
11 Profile of proprietor or partners including qualifications and experience in the field.
12 References.

Having prepared the business plan and arranged finance, the next stage will be to find the right premises. Once the premises have been found it will be necessary to contact a good solicitor to deal with all legal aspects, to keep the bank manager and accountant informed of progress, and then to contact the Local Authority planning department and environmental health office.

## Locating and organizing the right premises

Consideration should be given to the ease with which clients can reach the premises. Is public transport efficient and within easy reach? Will clients be able to park without difficulty? Look at the surrounding businesses – could they be an asset or might they have a detrimental effect, e.g. hairdressing or fashion could be beneficial, bringing clients into the area, whereas a public house or noisy record shop will have definite disadvantages!

Look at any existing businesses of a similar nature. Assess the competition – how many clients do they have? What is their price structure? Check the standard of treatments offered. Look into the size of the local population and decide whether the area can accommodate another practice.

There are two ways of obtaining business premises.

1  The property may be purchased outright by means of cash or business mortgage. Is the property freehold or leasehold? When the property is residential, check any restrictions concerning the use of the premises for business purposes. This is particularly valid if you are intending to use part of your home.
2  When purchasing the premium on a lease for an office or retail outlet, the details and restrictions of the lease should be studied very carefully, preferably by a solicitor. Is the lease a full repairing lease or will the landlord be responsible for repairs? What is the length of the lease, e.g. five years or more? How often is the rent reviewed?

### Planning department

Having found the right premises it may be necessary to contact the planning department of the Local Authority to apply for change of use. The planning department will want to know whether the property is in a residential area or located within a shopping area. If the area is residential will the proposed business cause aggravation to local residents? The Public Highways section will want to study the possible effect of increased traffic from clients. Will this cause a traffic hazard? Parking will be of prime consideration. Is parking within the immediate location sufficient to accommodate the number of people visiting the establishment?

### Environmental health department

The environmental health department will need to be satisfied that the following government acts are being observed:

1  Local Government (Miscellaneous Provisions) Act 1982;
2  Health and Safety at Work Act 1974;
3  Shops, Offices and Railway Premises Act 1963;
4  Electricity at Work Regulations 1990;
5  Fire Precautions Act 1971;
6  Control of Substances Hazardous to Health Regulations (COSHH).

*The Local Government (Miscellaneous Provisions) Act 1982* requires that any person carrying out electrical epilation should be registered with the Local Authority before commencing practice. It is the operator who must be registered, not the premises. Failure to register could result in a fine of up to £200.

An inspector from the environmental health department will visit the premises and communicate with the individual before issuing a certificate of registration. The inspector will wish to know about provisions for sanitation, hygiene, sterilization of equipment and instruments used. When needles are sterilized within the clinic, the inspector will wish to know the method used and whether it is effective. Many authorities will only accept the use of pre-sterilized disposable needles or the use of an autoclave. What procedure is followed for the disposal of contaminated needles? Storage of consumables such as bed rolls, cotton wool, tissues, antiseptic lotions, etc. will be noted.

The purpose of the *Health and Safety at Work Act 1974* is to secure the health, safety and welfare of both employees in the course of their work and self-employed persons throughout the time they devote to work.

The Act is also concerned with the protection of the individual against risks of health and safety arising out of, or in connection with, the activities of another person at work.

The employer's duty in relation to the Act is to ensure as far as is reasonably practicable the health, safety and welfare of his/her employees.

The employee's duty is to take reasonable care for the health and safety of him/herself, and of other persons who may be affected by his/her acts or omissions at work.

Offices, shops and railway premises are now regulated by the Health and Safety at Work Act 1974 and are therefore subject to the general provisions of that Act. Additionally, such premises may come within the scope of the *Offices, Shops and Railway Premises Act 1963.* This Act is restricted to premises in which persons are employed for a total of 21 hours or more per week. The Act does not apply to premises in which only self-employed persons work.

The section covering health, safety and welfare (general provisions) relates to cleanliness, overcrowding, temperature, ventilation, lighting, sanitary and washing facilities, etc., and to general provisions for first aid.

The section of the Act relating to fire precautions covers the provision of means of escape in case of fire, safety provisions in case of fire, certification of premises by the appropriate authority, fire alarms, fire prevention and provision of fire-fighting equipment.

The relevant Acts can be obtained from the reference section of the local lending library or can be purchased direct from Her Majesty's Stationery Office – address and telephone number will be found in the telephone directory.

*Fire regulations* must not be overlooked when opening a business. The local fire officer will visit the premises in order to inspect provisions in the way of fire extinguishers and exits from the building.

*The Fire Precautions Act 1977* states that all employees should be aware and trained in the emergency fire evacuation procedures. All members of staff should know where the nearest emergency exits are situated. These exits must be kept unlocked at all times during working hours. Staff should be aware of the fact that lifts must not be used in the event of fire or power failures, all personal belongings should be left behind, windows and doors

**Figure 20.1** Types of fire extinguisher

a) A *water* extinguisher for use on paper, wood textiles, and fabric. It must not be used on burning liquid, electrical or flammable metal fires

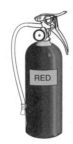

(b) A *foam* extinguisher for use on burning liquid fires. It must not be used on electrical or flammable metal fires

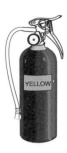

c) A *powder* extinguisher for use on burning liquid and electrical fires. It must not be used on flammable metal fires

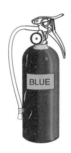

(d) A *halon* extinguisher for use on burning liquid and electrical fires. It must not be used on flammable metal fires

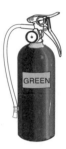

e) A *carbon dioxide* extinguisher for use on burning liquid and electrical fires. It must not be used on flammable metal fires

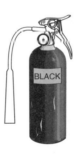

(f) A light-duty *fire* blanket for use on burning liquids and burning cloth. Heavy-duty fire blankets are available for industrial use

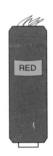

to be closed on leaving the premises wherever possible. Staff should also be aware of the location of fire appliances, the type of fire extinguishers, their uses and how to use them.

Both carbon dioxide (black) and water (red) fire extinguishers should be installed. Other extinguishers available are:

Powder (blue) for use on all types of fires.
Halon gas (green) for use on electrical fires.
Foam (yellow) for liquids.

They should be placed where they can be seen and reached easily in the event of a fire. It is advisable to have extinguishers serviced annually. Water extinguishers should not be used for electrical fires or near the mains supply. Carbon dioxide extinguishers can be used on all types of fire. A fire blanket is suitable for small fires. Exits should be clearly marked and free from obstructions.

Consumables such as paper bed rolls, tissues, cotton wool, surgical spirits, etc. should be stored away from any possible risk of fire, i.e. they should not be situated under or near the mains electricity supply. Magnifying lamps should be kept away from direct sunlight. When direct sunlight is concentrated through the lens on to a flammable material fire may result from the build-up of heat.

*The Electricity at Work Regulations Act 1990* states that all pieces of electrical equipment within the workplace should be checked annually by a qualified electrician, who will then label the equipment, stating the date of inspection.

### Additional basic legislation

### The Sale of Goods Act 1979

This Act states that goods offered must be fit for the purpose for which they are intended.

### Supply of Goods and Services Act

The purpose of this Act is to extend the protection given to consumers under the Sale of Goods Act to include services, goods on hire and goods given in exchange for gift vouchers.

### Trades Description Act 1968 and 1972

This Act states that the retailer must not give misleading information about goods and services, or make dishonest comparisons relating to prices to the consumer. Descriptions for both goods and services must be accurate.

### Control of Substances Hazardous to Health Regulations (COSHH) 1988

COSHH covers the storing and use of products containing hazardous substances, for example surgical spirit, hydrogen peroxide, chlorhexidine.

The regulations require that all products etc. which contain substances known to be hazardous to health are recorded with details of action to be taken in case of accidental exposure.

Specific symbols indicate the type of hazard for a particular substance. (See Figure 20.2.)

### Data Protection Act 1984

Computers are fast becoming an essential piece of office equipment in the clinic. It is now a legal requirement that when storing personal information (records) relating to clients the user should register with the Data Protection Registrar. Clients are now entitled to ask for copies of any information which has been stored and which concerns themselves. It is therefore important to appreciate that only information of a professional nature is recorded together with appointments etc. It is not wise to store any personal observations or comments. The application forms DPR1 or DPR4 (intended for use by small businesses) are available from:

The Data Protection Registrar,
Springfield House,
Water Lane,
Wilmslow,
Cheshire SK9 5AF
Tel: 01625-535-7777.

Holding of personal data on a computer by an unregistered person is a criminal offence.

**Figure 20.2**
Hazardous chemical
symbols

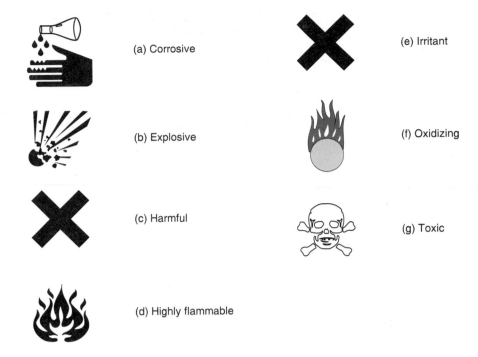

(a) Corrosive

(b) Explosive

(c) Harmful

(d) Highly flammable

(e) Irritant

(f) Oxidizing

(g) Toxic

## The role of computers in the clinic

Computers can prove to be an invaluable piece of equipment when chosen wisely and used correctly. They are ideal for keeping the business accounts, cash flow and profit forecasts, stock control, clients' records, treatment details and word processing.

Before buying a computer it is essential to decide exactly what the computer will be used for. Computers and their specifications change rapidly as does the software which is continually being upgraded. The upgrades usually require more hard disk space. Therefore before making the final purchase ensure that the model chosen will meet the needs of the clinic, that the hard disk is large enough to hold all the relevant information and that the software is suitable for the purpose for which it is intended. The most common mistake first time buyers make is to buy a computer that they will have outgrown within six months.

## Value Added Tax

VAT, or Value Added Tax, is levied on most business transactions that take place within the European Community (EC), the UK, and Isle of Man. This tax is called by different names and is of varying amounts in different countries. Each country is reponsible for its own rules and regulations relating to this tax. Her Majesty's Customs and Excise are responsible for the collection and administration of VAT in the UK.

It is a legal requirement for all businesses in the UK and Isle of Man to register with the VAT Office when trading turnover is likely to reach or exceed the threshold limit. The VAT threshold is set by the government and reassessed annually. The threshold limit in 1995 was set at £47,000 annual turnover. VAT is charged on taxable turnover, which is the value, not just the profit, of all taxable supplies made in the UK or

Isle of Man. Failure to register on time may result in the levying of a financial penalty. VAT returns should be completed and presented to the office at specified times, with financial penalties being imposed on late returns.

## Inland Revenue

The Inland Revenue will want to know the name of your accountant, the type of business you are running and whether you are a sole trader or in partnership.

At the end of each trading year, a copy of the business accounts should be sent to the tax inspector. Tax will be based on business income, less allowable business expenses. The accounts will need to satisfy the inspector that they show a true reflection of the business.

When taking on employees it may be necessary to deduct income tax and national insurance contributions from their earnings, as well as pay the employer's share of the national insurance contribution.

Employees normally pay income tax on the PAYE (pay as you earn) basis. The employer deducts tax from the employee's wages or salary each pay day and then pays the tax over to the Inland Revenue on a monthly basis. The tax year runs from 6 April one year to 5 April the following year.

It is essential to keep full and accurate records of business accounts for your own use, as well as for use by your accountant and the Inland Revenue. When registered, the VAT inspector may also ask to see the books.

Until January 1996 a self-employed person paid tax on the net taxable profits of the business on 1 January in the taxable year and on 1 July following the end of the tax year. The tax office notified the individual of the amount due.

In 1996 self-assessment was introduced by the Government. The *Finance Act 1994* contains the main legislation for a major reform of the taxation system. It affects all taxpayers who have to submit a tax return including self-employed individuals, business partners, company directors, employees who pay tax at the higher rate, together with other employees and pensioners with reasonably complex tax affairs.

The term 'self assessment' can be misleading. The Inland Revenue has the power to amend obvious errors in tax returns and to carry out in depth enquiries where appropriate. They also have the authority to make random selection of tax returns for more detailed examination and closed years may be re-opened where the Inland Revenue have evidence that tax returns are incorrect or incomplete.

Employees who do not normally fill in a tax return continue to pay tax under the PAYE system.

By careful planning of accounting dates, useful cashflow advantages can be obtained in the early years of a growing business.

## National insurance contributions

National insurance contributions are paid by all employed and self-employed persons unless exemption has been granted.

For employees, deductions will be made direct from salary by the employer, along with income tax on the PAYE basis. These are class 1 national insurance contributions and are liable when earnings reach a lower earning limit. The amount deducted will be earnings-related. Contributions will be made by both the employer and the employee.

When sufficient contributions have been made the employee will be entitled to claim for sickness and invalidity benefit, unemployment benefit, widow's benefit and maternity allowance. A portion of contributions goes towards the retirement pension.

When self-employed, weekly class 2 national insurance contributions should be paid either by stamping a card every week or by direct debit through the bank. These weekly contributions will be paid at a flat rate regardless of earnings. At the end of the tax year a further earnings-related class 4 contribution may be required based on a percentage of the taxable profit of the business.

Benefits available to the self-employed are basic sickness and invalidity benefits, and basic maternity allowance. A contribution will be made to the basic retirement pension.

Full information relating to national insurance contributions can be obtained from the local employment office and the Department of Social Security. The telephone numbers will be in the local telephone directory.

## Costing of treatments

This is an area that is often neglected. The temptation is to undercut the local competition without sufficient thought to the future. It is very difficult to increase prices in a short period of time if you get the pricing structure wrong.

The treatment fee should reflect the overheads, costs, and an allowance for profit margin. Psychology also plays a part in the pricing of treatments. Should the price charged be too low, the client will have little confidence in the therapist's ability. When the price is too high and does not reflect value for money the client will look elsewhere.

The trading costs for a 12 month period should be looked at in detail. These include rent, rates, electricity, heating, lighting, replacement and maintenance of equipment, consumables such as needles, cotton wool, paper bed rolls, tissues etc, wages, telephone, advertising costs, stationery and printing costs, insurances, and accountancy fees.

The number of trading hours available should be considered and allowances made for bank holidays and traditionally quiet periods such as January and February and perhaps October. An assessment of the overheads and running costs can be made from the above, and a realistic treatment fee arrived at.

## Choosing suppliers

Reliable and efficient suppliers of both equipment and consumables are an asset to any well-run business.

When looking for equipment check that it is safe, well made, reliable and will do the required job. Then enquire into delivery dates, service and repair facilities and whether or not the supplier offers a back-up service should it be necessary.

When choosing suppliers for consumables look to see if there is a good cash and carry in the area. If so, are the premises easy to get to? How do the trading hours compare with those of the proposed business? If you are considering use of mail order, find out how efficient is the service offered.

167

How much is charged for goods supplied through the service? Is the quality of goods up to the standard required? Are the goods readily available when they are needed?

A good working relationship with the right supplier can be of great value to the business.

## Choosing equipment

When buying equipment a number of points need to be considered before making the final decision:

- Is the equipment going to used in the salon and therefore remains in one position or is to be used in a mobile practice?
- Is the equipment safe?
- Is the equipment well-made, reliable and durable?
- Enquire into delivery dates, service and repair facilities.
- Does the supplier offer a back-up service ?
- Does the price reflect the quality of the equipment?
- Make certain that the equipment has been manufactured in accordance with current European regulations (EU countries only).

## Maintenance of equipment

Equipment should be serviced regularly and checked by an electrician annually (see the Electricity at Work Regulations Act, page 164).

In addition the following maintenance procedures should be followed as a matter of routine:

- Check plugs, leads and wires to ensure there are no loose connections.
- Equipment should be cleaned daily.
- Check regularly for wear and tear.
- Epilation machines should be kept on a suitable trolley during use.
- Castors on trolleys and stools should be looked at to ensure they are working efficiently and are not broken or loose.
- Electrical leads and wires should not be allowed to trail on the floor.
- Always check that the machine is working correctly before commencing treatments.

## Insurance

Insurance is an essential consideration when setting up in business. The hope is that a claim will never be necessary, yet realistically no business or practising therapist can afford to be without adequate cover. Who knows what may happen in the future – possibly through no fault of your own!

Some policies are required by law, e.g. car insurance, employer's liability when employing staff.

There are a number of policies that can be considered when setting up in practice, some of which are necessary or advisable, while others can be added at a later date when funds permit.

*Treatment risk* protects the therapist against legal liability for accidental injury or damage to a client arising out of treatment, e.g. scars from incorrect electrical epilation, injury to an eye, or permanent damage which may result in psychological distress. The onus is on the client to prove that the injury or damage suffered is due to the fault of the therapist.

*Employer's liability* is a legal requirement when employing staff. This policy covers the employer for legal liability in the event of injury to an employee arising out of their employment.

*Public liability* covers the therapist for accidental loss or damage to property and for accidental injury to any person arising in connection with the business. For example a customer may trip on a defective carpet in the therapist's premises and sue for damages.

*Building and contents* should be covered against fire, flooding, storm damage, gales, burglary, theft and other specified perils. This type of insurance can be extended to include accidental damage. The extension is more expensive due to the increased risk.

*Business interruption.* The policy covers interruption to business following a disaster such as fire, flood, storm, etc. and extends to include denial of access and failure of public utilities.

*Car insurance premiums* will be higher when a car is used in connection with business. It is necessary to inform the insurance company that cover for business use is required, and failure to do so may result in the insurance company refusing to meet any claim that arises when the car is being used for this purpose.

*Permanent health insurance* provides long-term protection for loss of income arising through illness, injury or accident. When self-employed, illness or permanent disability can result in serious financial hardship. Commitments such as mortgage, community charge, electricity, gas, telephone and food still have to be met.

Statutory sick pay, sickness benefit and invalidity benefit provided by the government are designed only to protect against poverty and do not provide sufficient income to maintain standards of living. The premium for permanent health insurance will vary, depending on the amount of benefit required, whether there is a deferment period of four weeks or more before benefit may be claimed, and the general state of health of the person insured.

*General personal accident insurance* pays specific benefits (e.g. death, loss of eye or limbs) due to injury following an accident, provided that the cause is not connected with high-risk activities such as winter sports. This cover does not include illness of any type. *Hand disablement* covers just the hands below the wrist and includes illness and accident, e.g. broken finger or contracted dermatitis.

It is wise to contact a registered insurance broker for advice concerning the relevant policies. Registered insurance brokers are able to recommend the most suitable policy for your individual needs. They know which insurance companies are reliable.

## Advertising and public relations

When setting up in business, advertising and public relations are two valuable aids that can play a major role in attracting clients.

*Advertising* when used correctly can encourage prospective clients to make contact for further information, or to book a consultation. The purpose is to let people know about you, your qualifications, the services offered and the location of the clinic, or practice and to provide a contact number. In other words the aim is to inform people of your existence and encourage them through the door.

For an advertisement to be effective it must be:

1 well set out and displayed;
2 carefully and honestly worded;
3 informative but to the point;
4 tasteful and eye-catching.

In other words it must state clearly what you want to say, without cramming too much information into a limited space. A small advertisement, placed on a regular basis in a prominent position is more effective than a large, expensive display that appears once only.

An *advertisement feature* taking a quarter- to half-page in the local newspaper can be a good introduction and catch the public's eye. Half the feature could be in the form of an editorial. This is a way of bringing you, your establishment and the services offered, to the attention of many prospective clients. Indeed it has been known for future clients to keep a feature such as this and telephone for an appointment several *months* later.

A feature of this kind should be followed by the insertion of several smaller, yet well-placed advertisements in the same newspaper. Fortnightly insertions are sometimes more effective than weekly appearances. When people take it for granted that your advertisement will always appear there is no urgency to make contact, but its sudden disappearance can provide the jolt that stimulates the client into action.

Positioning is of vital importance. The advertisement stands more chance of being noticed if it is placed at the top right-hand corner of the right-hand page. It comes into view as soon as the page is opened. Front and back pages are also desirable positions, as is the women's page. When a client is specifically looking for the services of an electrolysist she may turn to the yellow pages or to the classified section of the paper under 'Health and Beauty'. When placed in the classified section a boxed advertisement with a bold outline will stand out, and will catch the eye. Be careful about advertising in the personal column, which can give the wrong impression – it depends on the quality and standards of the newspaper concerned.

**Figure 20.3** Example of an advertisement

*Mrs Godfrey*

DRE, FBAE, BABTAC

International specialist in

**ELECTROLYSIS**

Treatment for the removal of unwanted hair and broken capillaries using disposable sterile needles

For details and confidential consultation without obligation contact:

**The Electrolysis Clinic**
79 Westbrook Road, Four Oaks, West Midlands B29 1QZ
Tel: 01564 060791

Incorrect positioning can be a complete waste of time and money. The advertisement must be placed in a prominent position. Timing is also important. Money is wasted if advertisements are inserted just before Christmas, bank holidays and traditionally quiet times of the year.

For the electrolysist in private practice, who is mobile or running a small-to medium-sized clinic, the use of television or glossy magazines is not cost-effective. The expense is high for very little return.

Local businesses such as hairdressers, fashion outlets and hotels are often happy to leave your business card on display. Contact should be made through the proprietor or manager.

Plan your advertising campaign with care and allocate a budget for this purpose. In the early days when clients are few, carefully planned and placed advertising can more than pay for itself. As the number of clients increase the need for advertising decreases.

*Public relations* is all about promoting the business through image, and presentation, and through making contact, both socially and professionally, with key people in the locality.

The business premises should be warm, with a welcoming atmosphere and should at the same time portray a professional image. The décor should be subtle, encouraging relaxation. The surroundings should appear clean and hygienic without being too clinical. The ambiance should be one that encourages clients to enter the premises, book an appointment and return for further treatment.

The personal appearance of the electrolysist and staff will make an immediate impact on the client. Untidy hair, heavy or bizarre make-up, long enamelled nails, scruffy uniform, laddered stockings and dirty shoes do not give a favourable impression. A well-groomed appearance and pleasant manner will do much to create the right impression. Teaming this with expertise and knowledge of subject is a sure way to gain new clients.

Successful public relations can be achieved in many ways:

1  free editorial in local newspaper;
2  letter of introduction to local GPs and key medical personnel;
3  lectures to local organizations;
4  hospital work;
5  open days or evenings;
6  guest appearances on local television programmes;
7  radio phone-ins;
8  leaflets in dental waiting rooms.

Taking each of the above points in turn, how can they be achieved?

Unwanted hair causes distress and embarrassment to many people. The features editor of the women's page in the local paper may be interested in writing an article on the subject. It helps if you already advertise with the paper. Ring the editor and introduce yourself. Arrange a meeting to discuss the subject. Before the meeting make sure you have all the relevant information to hand, with the important facts in writing – this helps to ensure that the facts are taken down correctly. If the editor is not familiar with electrical epilation offer to write the article yourself. In this way you can ensure that the details are accurate. Be prepared to promote yourself and your business, while maintaining the professional image.

Send a letter of introduction to local doctors, particularly those in private practice, gynaecologists, endocrinologists and dermatologists. The letter should include details of your experience, qualifications, membership of relevant professional associations and where you practise. Remember to keep it short and to the point.

Liaise with the client's doctor when necessary, but do *not* waste his/her time with trivial matters. Referrals should state the name and address of the client and the nature of the problem, together with brief details of intended treatment.

Lectures to local organizations such as luncheon clubs, Women's Institutes, Townswomen's Guild and Inner Wheel are a good way of introducing the subject of electrical epilation to many people who may wish to know more but lack the confidence to ask. Often it is a case of not knowing who to go to for treatment or how to find out! The audience at such meetings will be listening and looking at you for at least 30 to 45 minutes. This is an ideal opportunity to promote yourself and your knowledge while creating the right impression.

Hospital work on a voluntary basis can be most satisfying, as well as a means of establishing valuable contacts. Second-year students in the beauty department of a well-known and respected college of technology have for many years run a voluntary cosmetic camouflage clinic at the local hospital. All those involved have benefitted. The patients gained from the help they were given in camouflaging their disfigurements; the students by their increased knowledge and experience; and the college by referrals for electrical epilation many of whom could not afford to pay privately for treatment. Those who attended the college for electrical epilation did so knowing that all classes were fully supervized by experienced, qualified tutors.

An open day or evening which brings people into the premises often creates interest. An effective way of encouraging people through the door is to turn the event into a fund-raising function. People are far more inclined to attend when they are supporting a local charity, or contributing towards specific equipment for a local hospital.

A guest appearance on a local radio phone-in or television programme is a good way of introducing the subject of electrical epilation to the general public. Make contact by ringing the presenters of suitable programmes. These people are always looking for interesting subject matter. Although programmes will not mention specific clinics it will be possible to give the name and address of the professional associations concerned with electrical epilation. Interested parties will then contact the association, who in turn will pass on your name – provided that you are a member!

## Consultation/record cards

The consultation/record card should contain all relevant details concerning each client. Information to be recorded includes:

- medical history and any prescribed medications;
- menstrual cycle, irregularities and number of pregnancies;

- possible cause of hair growth;
- previous treatment if applicable;
- length and frequency of previous treatments;
- presence of pigmentation marks or scars;
- temporary methods of hair removal used;
- skin type and healing rate.

Treatment records should include:

- date and length of treatment session;
- method of electro-epilation used, together with intensity of currents;
- needle size, texture of hair and area treated;
- skin reaction to treatment.

Accurately recorded details of treatment enable the operator to monitor treatment progress together with alterations in hair growth pattern and distribution. This in turn will enable the operator to determine future treatment requirements according to the client's needs.

## Telephone enquiries and bookings

The telephone often forms the first point of contact between the clinic and the prospective client. Clients may be nervous or know very little about electro-epilation when making the inital enquiry.

During this telephone conversation the receptionist or electrolysist should evaluate the person's problem and explain the procedure and purpose of electro-epilation. Information regarding the value of a clinic consultation should be given.

The name and address of the enquirer can be taken so that details of electro-epilation may be sent through the post if desired. The advantage of forwarding details of the clinic and treatment procedure is that it enables the recipient to read the relevant information prior to the initial consultation.

The receptionist/electrolysist should have a warm, pleasant telephone manner and a clear voice. The caller should not be kept waiting on an open line. It is irritating to the caller and leads to dissatisfaction. When booking appointments over the telephone state the date, time and day of the appointment clearly and then confirm by repeating these details.

At times it may be necessary to use the facilities of an answerphone. In this situation the outgoing message should be clear and any messages received should be dealt with at the earliest opportunity.

## Receptionist

The receptionist plays a key role in the smooth running of the salon. It is the receptionist who provides the initial point of contact and is usually the first person the client sees or talks to when entering the salon.

The receptionist should be friendly, professional and welcoming without being over familiar. The client must be made to feel welcome and at ease.

It is an advantage for the receptionist to be familiar with epilation treatment and be able to explain the procedure when a prospective client makes a general enquiry. The receptionist should encourage the person concerned to attend for an initial consultation with one of the electrolosists.

The receptionist should have the ability to deal with all manner of people without becoming flustered, harassed, argumentative or intolerant.

## Review questions

1 Define the term 'business plan'.
2 Why is it advisable to draw up a business plan prior to setting up in business?
3 List the points to be considered when choosing the location for an electro-epilation practice.
4 What is covered by the Health and Safety at Work Act 1974?
5 Name two different types of fire extinguisher and state what type of fire each would be used on.
6 What do the initials VAT stand for?
7 Who is responsible for collecting VAT in the UK?
8 How do employees normally pay income tax?
9 Why is it necessary to keep a full and accurate record of all business accounts?
10 What are national insurance contributions and why are they paid?
11 List the benefits of national insurance contributions to:
   (a) an employee
   (b) a self-employed person.
12 State the points that should be considered when costing treatments.
13 Name and describe three different insurance policies that should be taken out when starting in business.
14 Explain the difference between advertising and public relations.
15 Name four ways in which successful public relations can be achieved.
16 Explain the importance of keeping accurate, up-to-date record cards.
17 Describe the procedure that should be followed when taking a telephone booking.

# 21 Professional ethics

The term 'professional ethics' refers to the code of conduct, or standards of behaviour practised by the professional electrolysist in relation to:

- clients
- colleagues
- the medical profession
- the professional association of which the electrolysist is a member

Courtesy, honesty and integrity are all essential qualities which separate the caring professionals from the cowboys.

## Ethics concerning clients

At all times clients should receive caring, professional treatment. Honest information should be given in relation to duration and progress of treatment. False promises, or prolonged treatment for financial gain will be far from beneficial with regard to the electrolysist's long-term reputation.

The client should be able to expect and receive total confidentiality at all times; nor should information concerning one client be discussed with another. Conversations involving controversial subjects such as religion, politics and racial matters are best avoided.

Clients' appointments, once made, should not be cancelled or altered by the electrolysist without good reason. There are times when an event such as illness, a death in the family or a major crisis may prevent the electrolysist from keeping appointments and in such situations clients must be notified in advance to prevent wasted journeys and possible ill-feeling. The majority of clients are understanding in such circumstances.

The appointment book should be organized to allow for accurate time-keeping so that clients are not kept waiting. To run late occasionally is acceptable and inevitable; to do so on a regular basis shows inefficient organization and lack of courtesy towards the clients.

Many clients are inclined to talk about their personal problems during treatment. The electrolysist is often the only person they can talk to about such matters. It is essential that any such conversation takes place in total confidence and is *never* discussed with a third party. In these circumstances the electrolysist should not offer personal advice, since this could give rise to a number of difficulties at a later date.

The client's best interests should always be of prime consideration.

## Ethics concerning colleagues

A true professional does not attempt to poach clients from colleagues, and does not speak disparagingly about another electrolysist's standard of work.

Occasions arise when an electrolysist will attend to a colleague's clients on a temporary basis, for example during holiday periods or times of ill-health. When this situation occurs the original treatment plan should not be altered in any way without consultation with the colleague concerned.

A minority of clients exist who tend to flit from one clinic to another, or who make appointments with two electrolysists. Once this situation has been brought to the attention of either operator it must not be allowed to continue, in order to safeguard the electrolysist concerned and to prevent the client's skin from receiving too much treatment. Such a situation prevents accurate record-keeping of treatment progress.

## Ethics concerning the medical profession

Clients expect electrolysists to be able to recognize and pass opinon on any number of skin conditions and medically related matters. It is well known that many skin lesions demonstrate similar characteristics, some of which may be benign, whereas others may be malignant, but it is not for the electrolysist to decide. Electrolysists should pass comment only on subjects in which they are professionally qualified. There will be instances in which no treatment should be given without first obtaining written agreement from a medical practitioner.

The electrolysist's work can be divided into three categories: those which cover cosmetic purposes; those which are hormone related but do not require medical liaison, e.g. menopause; and those for which medical referral is necessary.

The initial consultation may indicate the possible existence of a condition which requires medical investigation prior to electro-epilation, or an established disorder such as diabetes or epilepsy. In such circumstances consultation with the client's GP will be necessary before any treatment can be given.

It is essential that an electrolysist knows when to refer clients to the medical profession. Equally, busy doctors soon become irritated by unnecessary communication on irrelevant matters. Where a medical practitioner agrees to electro-epilation treatment, progress reports can be sent to that practitioner as and when necessary. This not only keeps the doctor informed but also helps to build a good working relationship between the medical and electrolysis professions.

## Professional associations

The two associations in the UK concerned purely with electro-epilation are:

1  the British Association of Electrolysists Ltd;
2  the Institute of Electrolysis.

Both have similar aims and objectives, which are primarily concerned with promoting the professional status of electrolysis.

Membership of a professional association by the practising electrolysist may soon be of paramount importance. The full implications of 1992 concerning matters relating to training standards, professional qualifications, and the removal of trade barriers within the EC are not yet known.

Membership of an association provides many benefits for the practising electrolysist including:

1  lectures and demonstrations;
2  meetings which allow the interchange of ideas between colleagues;
3  members of the general public do contact the associations for a list of qualified practitioners;

4   promotion of electrolysis through publicity in national magazines, newspapers and reference libraries;
5   refresher and advanced epilation courses through the association's lists of recognized tutors.

The associations, quite rightly, expect members to maintain high professional standards and to adhere to their codes of conduct. Each association holds an annual general meeting at which all business matters and information relating to the running of the association are presented to the membership. It is often surprising how few members make the effort to attend these meetings. Presumably those who do not attend are happy with the way their association is being run by their elected council!

It is the author's opinion that any electrolysist who is serious about his/her career will not only gain many benefits from belonging to a professional association, but by taking an active part will also be able to make a valuable contribution to the profession as a whole.

For those students and qualified practitioners who are interested in contacting or becoming a member, a list of professional associations and contact addresses is given at the end of this book.

# 22 Case histories

The following case histories relate to clients who have attended the author's clinic with successful results:

**Case history 1**

A 58-year-old woman with heavy growth of terminal hair on chin, neck, jaw line and upper lip, attended for an initial consultation. Previous treatment with an unqualified operator had proved unsuccessful, and this client was somewhat disenchanted with electro-epilation. However, desperation concerning her problem led her to try again, this time having obtained a list of qualified practitioners from the Institute of Electrolysis.

The initial consultation revealed surgery for the removal of fibroids and abscesses from the womb. There was no history of menstrual irregularity or hormonal disturbance other than those associated with menopause, which had not caused undue problems. The cause appeared to be genetic predisposition relating to sensitivity of follicles to circulating androgens. Mechanical interference included regular waxing and tweezing.

The client was adamant that she wanted to attend for treatment on a daily basis. A compromise was reached of 20-minute sessions three times weekly, working in rotation on chin, upper lip and jaw line. In this way the client was given peace of mind, yet each area was allowed sufficient healing time prior to further treatment. Had the client not been allowed to attend so regularly there is no doubt she would have attended two clinics for treatment without keeping either informed of what she was doing. Psychology had a large part to play in the treatment of this client.

Blend treatment was the method chosen for chin, neck and jaw line with shortwave diathermy being used on the upper lip. During the course of treatment it was noted that regrowth was considerably less on the areas where blend had been used. Treatment sessions were for 20 minutes, three times weekly for six months, dropping to twice weekly for five weeks, then weekly thereafter. Appointments gradually became less frequent as the condition improved. A successful result was achieved over a period of 20 months.

During this period the client's attitude and personality changed from being aggressive, rude and argumentative, to pleasant and outgoing with a lively sense of humour. Self-esteem improved, together with a remarkable change in appearance. This client joined Weight Watchers, and lost 15 kilos, had her hair restyled and took far more interest in clothes. Her husband was delighted with the change in his wife, but to this day, some five years later, is still unaware of why the change occurred.

**Case history 2**

A lady aged 61 years with one son aged 26 had a problem with excessive hair growth that had started at the age of 17 after she had received progesterone injections. This client lacked confidence and was shy and reserved. The areas affected involved the sides of the face, chin, jaw line and upper lip. The client spent 25 minutes on a daily basis waxing and tweezing. The client's son, aware of his mother's distress, contacted the British Association of Electrolysis for advice and a list of qualified electrolysists.

Initial treatment was given with shortwave diathermy in order to clear the area quickly, using a size 004 needle. Duration of treatment was 45 minutes per week. After four weeks treatment was changed to weekly sessions of one hour using blend. Over a period of 13 months the length of sessions gradually reduced to 15 minutes, and the needle size changed from 004 to 003 and finally 002. The length and frequency of treatments were determined by the appearance of regrowth. Treatment was completed after a period of 25 months.

When this client first attended for treatment she would rush into the clinic and found it difficult to look any member of staff in the eye. Her self-confidence was nil, and her life revolved around her son. As her hair growth problem decreased she became more outgoing and interested in life, taking up golf as a hobby. She has since recommended several of her friends to the clinic for treatment. Her words on more than one occasion have been 'Electrolysis has changed my life – I cannot believe the difference it has made to me. No longer having to wax and tweeze on a daily basis has given me a new lease of life.'

## Case history 3

This case history concerns a 19-year-old university student. She first attended the clinic at the age of 16, with fine, soft dark hair on the upper lip, which caused a shadow. This was treated with shortwave diathermy using a size 003 needle, thinning out the number of hairs present. Ten sessions of 15 minutes duration given at two- to three-weekly intervals achieved a successful result. This client returned three years later in distress. She had gained weight steadily, coarse hair growth had appeared in a masculine pattern on the face, and acne type lesions were present. The skin had become excessively oily, and menstruation was irregular. This client was referred to her GP initially, who in turn sent her to a gynaecologist.

Stein-Leventhal syndrome (polycystic ovaries) was diagnosed. Treatment involved hormone therapy in conjunction with blend treatment over a period of nine months. This particular situation was diagnosed and dealt with at the early stages of development. Consequently hormone therapy was able to deal with the underlying cause relatively quickly and electro-epilation dealt with existing hair growth that had not been aggravated by mechanical interference. Blend was given at fortnightly intervals for 30 minutes during the university holidays only. Treatment was completed in 15 months.

## Case history 4

A 17-year-old student attended for treatment to two small patches of sparse coarse hair on either side of the chin. The growth had appeared just after puberty, since which time the client had plucked regularly. Follicles were distorted and the skin sensitive to treatment by shortwave diathermy. There were no menstrual irregularities or history of genetic predisposition to hypertrichosis. Treatment was given every three weeks initially, using size 004 needle and later changing to size 003.

During the following three years noticeable hair growth began to appear in a masculine pattern on the face, sternum, breast, abdomen and thighs.

**Case history 4 – continued**

The client was referred to her GP who was unsympathetic and refused to send her to a specialist. The client eventually changed to another practitioner who recommended a skin specialist, who in turn referred her to an endocrinologist. Eventually Stein-Leventhal syndrome was diagnosed. The procedure had taken two and a half years from the first appointment with the original doctor to the final diagnosis by the endocrinologist. During this time electro-epilation, using shortwave diathermy, was given fortnightly to try to keep the facial hair growth under control.

Once the cause of the problem had been diagnosed, hormone therapy was prescribed for 18 months, the client attending the specialist every six months. During the course of hormone therapy the body hair growth became finer, softer in texture and less noticeable. Established facial hair responded well to blend treatment in conjunction with the hormone therapy. The needle size was gradually reduced from 004 to 002. Initially, weekly appointments were given, with the time between treatments gradually increasing as the condition improved.

The course of treatment for this client was a prolonged one, spanning some five years from start to finish. Although the cause of the problem was exactly the same as for the client in the previous case history, the results were slower due to the length of time taken to reach a diagnosis. In the first instance the client's GP was sympathetic and acted quickly, which meant that remedial treatment was started at the early stages, whereas the second client had to fight hard for referral to the right specialist, therefore treatment was delayed for two and a half years.

**Case history 5**

A 27-year-old woman was distressed by the presence of dark, coarse hair growth on the chin and neck, that had first appeared 10 years before. Medical investigation had revealed no endocrine abnormalities but a hyper-sensitization of the hair follicles to circulating androgens in the bloodstream. Stress aggravated the condition. Electro-epilation was recommended by her specialist as the only suitable method of treatment. This client had been plucking hairs on a daily basis for several years. She was very inhibited, embarrassed and difficult to engage in conversation. For the first few treatment sessions she would not attend without her mother being present.

The skin did not respond well to shortwave diathermy, and distorted follicles were present, so blend became the chosen method of treatment. Treatment sessions commenced with 45 minutes on a weekly basis, using a 005 needle. A galvanic setting of 0.5 ma and a high-frequency setting of 2 ma were used, with an average of six seconds blended current application followed by two seconds of galvanic after-count. Cataphoresis was applied at the end of each session. The needle size was gradually reduced to 002 and treatment sessions to 15 minutes, with the frequency of appointments reducing as the condition improved. Treatment was spread over a 16-month period.

During her course of treatment this client became less inhibited and started a teacher training course. She was delighted with her new-found confidence and change of career.

**Case history 6**

This client was a 49-year-old magistrate who had noticed the appearance of dark hair on the upper lip and chin, corresponding with the start of irregular periods, when she was 47. Hair had been removed regularly by waxing or tweezing. Growth was of medium texture, with distorted follicles. The client did not need hormone replacement therapy and was not being prescribed any form of medication. Treatment was successfully carried out over an 11-month period using blend. Initially, 20-minute sessions were given on a weekly basis, then fortnightly, progressing to three visits during the final three months.

This small sample of case histories shows that no two clients are alike, even though the underlying cause of the problem may be the same. Clients vary in their response and commitment to treatment. Every course of treatment must be tailored to suit the needs of the individual, with the client's long-term well-being and best interests being of prime consideration.

# National and Scottish Vocational Qualification Level 3

The National and Scottish Vocational Qualifications are aimed at encouraging a closer link between industry and education. Theses qualifications are based on standards developed by Industry and Commerce with the purpose of raising standards of competence while giving individuals recognition for their skills.

N/SVQs are available through centres approved by awarding bodies which have been accredited by the National Council for Vocational Qualifications.

Each qualification is broken down into units. Each unit encompasses several elements. In Electrical Epilation Level 3 there are five core units which must be completed, in addition to the specialist Epilation units.

To achieve a N/SVQ, students must successfully complete a wide range of specified work-based assessments. As far as possible an assessor will observe students in their usual workplace, carrying out normal work related activities. When this is not possible the assessment will take place in a simulated work situation which has been set up to relate as closely as possible to the normal working environment.

A key feature of N/SVQs is that they are qualifications about 'work' and any assessment of the candidate's competence will need to be based on his/her ability to perform competently in the workplace.

## Core units

To gain an N/SVQ in Level 3 Electrical Epilation the following five units must be obtained:

BO4*  Undertake salon reception duties.
BO17* Handling stock.
CO1   Assess the client for treatment.
CO2   Maintain services and operations to meet quality standards.
DO3   Contribute to the planning, monitoring and control of resources.

* These units are transferable from Level 2/3.

There is one specialist unit in electrical epilation:

DO1   Provide diathermy needle epilation.

There is also an additional unit available for those who wish to practise the Blend or galvanic electrolysis:

DO2   Provide galvanic/high frequency 'blend' epilation.

# DO1 Provide diathermy needle epilation

This unit is broken down into five elements:

**Element 1  Maintain standards of hygiene relating to personal and professional**

This element covers hair, nails, hands, feet, uniform equipment/materials – towels, couch covers, containers etc.

**Element 2  Prepare client plan for diathermy needle epilation**

This second element covers the consultation procedure and technique, as well as treatment planning.

The following points are noted during assessment. Is the student's approach to the client sensitive and caring? What is the technique for gaining the following information:

Skin analysis, medical background, history of the problem. Assessment of client – personality, relaxed, nervous, aggressive etc.

Area to be treated. Texture, type and density of hair growth.

Analysis of consultation – analysing the information gained during the consultation to enable the candidate to work out a suitable treatment plan for the client.

**Element 3 Provide diathermy needle epilation**

This section covers the practical application of treatment together with the care and comfort of the client. The student should be able to prepare the area for treatment and demonstrate the removal of hair from the following areas:

- Face.
- Arms.
- Breasts.
- Legs.

Treatment should be demonstrated on clients of differing temperament, age, lifestyle. Students will also be expected to know the structure and function of the skin, contra-indications to treatment and interpretation of body language.

The importance of discussing effectiveness of treatment together with the cost and proposed treatment plan should not be overlooked.

Students should also be able to explain the importance of establishing the client's lifestyle, physical and emotional condition, previous treatment, and any reactions.

**Element 4 Applying diathermy needle epilation**

This element looks into the practical application of epilation in relation to the correct type and size of needle, together with the maintenance of hygiene procedures during the treatment.

Current intensity, duration of current application to the follicle, spacing of treatment and the ease in which hair epilates from the follicle. The hair should slide out easily without traction or undue discomfort to the client.

Disposal of hairs and sharps would be covered in this element.

**Element 5
Aftercare**

The final element in this unit encompasses the accuracy and legibility of record cards, and the treatment plan and any changes which have been made to the original treatment plan.

Other points covered at this stage would be information on management of hair growth between clinic treatments and the explanation of aftercare to the client.

## DO2 Provide galvanic/high frequency 'Blend' needle epilation – additional unit

Elements 1 to 3 cover the same subject matter as elements 1 to 3 in diathermy needle epilation.

Element 4, in addition to the practical aspects covering diathermy needle epilation, the following should be included:

- During Blend treatment the passive electrode should be held by the client.
- Correct ratio and balance of the two currents during blend treatment.
- Principles and procedures for calculating the current ration of high frequency and galvanic currents. Application time of currents, current intensities, skin reaction, client comfort.
- Galvanic burns – recognition and treatment procedure.

Element 5 provides aftercare for high-frequency and galvanic 'Blend' needle epilation.

The purpose of the National/Scottish Vocational qualifications is to enable individuals to gain a work-based qualification through continual assessment without the disadvantages and stresses of one final examination which may take place in artificial conditions.

The Health and Beauty Therapy Training Board (HBTTB) is the leading body responsible for setting the standards for beauty therapy and epilation and at present is reviewing the existing standards to ensure they continue to reflect the needs of industry.

**Study Guide for N/SVQ Level 3 Electrical Epilation**

| Chapter | CO1 | CO2 | CO3 | Unit BO4 | B17 | DO1 | DO2 |
|---------|-----|-----|-----|----------|-----|-----|-----|
| 1 | | | | | | X | |
| 2 | | | | | | X | |
| 3 | | | | | | X | |
| 4 | | | | | | X | |
| 5 | | | | | | X | |
| 6 | | | | | | X | |
| 7 | | | | | | X | |
| 8 | | | | | | X | |
| 9 | | | | | | X | |
| 10 | | | | | | X | |
| 11 | | | | | | | X |
| 12 | | | | | | X | |
| 13 | | | | | | | X |
| 14 | | | | | | X | |
| 15 | X | | | | | X | |
| 16 | X | | | | | X | |
| 17 | | | | | | | |
| 18 | X | | | | | X | X |
| 19 | | | | | | X | X |
| 20 | | X | X | X | X | | |
| 21 | | X | X | | | | |

# Glossary

**Adrenal glands** are situated one above each kidney. They produce a number of hormones which include adrenalin (US name *epinephrine*) and steroids.

**Advertising** the aim of advertising is to inform people of services and products available.

**Acid mantle** a fine acidic film of sebum and sweat found on the surface of the skin. Its function is to inhibit the growth of bacteria.

**Acne** due to a defect in the sebaceous glands which leads to over production of sebum. It is primarily androgen induced and may indicate hypersensitization of sebaceous glands to circulating hormones.

**AIDS** (acquired immune deficiency syndrome) which develops as a result of infection by the human immune deficiency virus.

**Allergy** hyper sensitivity to a substance which causes the body to react to any contact with it in an adverse manner.

**Anagen** active stage of hair growth, where lower follicle is rebuilt and new hair is formed.

**Anorexia nervosa** psychological disorder, characterized by fear of becoming fat and refusal of food. Normally affects young adolescent girls. Involves the nervous, endocrine and digestive systems.

**Antiseptic** chemical which inhibits or destroys the growth of microorganisms on living tissue.

**Aseptic** free from organisms capable of causing disease.

**Asexual hair** growth not governed by hormones, e.g. scalp, eyebrows, eyelashes.

**Autoclave** piece of equipment used to sterilize instruments by steam at temperatures in excess of 100 centigrade.

**Benign** harmless. Non-cancerous.

**Blend epilation** the application of direct current and high frequency to the hair follicle simultaneously.

**Boil** staphylococcal infection of the hair follicle.

**Catagen** second stage of hair follicle growth cycle. Follows anagen. Hair separates from dermal papilla; club hair is formed. Lower follicle begins to shrivel and collapse.

**Club hair** develops during catagen. The bulk of the hair dries out and becomes brush-like. The club hair is held in the follicle by the cells of the inner root sheath.

**Cauterization** occurs when a high intensity of high frequency is passed into the tissue. Moisture vaporizes and tissue becomes dry.

**Chemical depilatories** chemical preparations which are applied to the skin in order to dissolve the hair. Temporary method of hair removal.

**Chloasma** patches of increased pigmentation, usually seen on the face during pregnancy. It may also occur during the menopause.

**Comedone** collection of sebum, keratinized cells and certain waste substances which accumulate in the entrance of a hair follicle.

**Consultation**   the initial meeting between client and electrolysist, which should form the basis of a professional relationship.

**Contra-indication**   the presence of any condition which indicates, or shows that electrical epilation should not be carried out.

**Cross-infection**   the transfer of infection from one person to another.

**Dermis**   lies under the epidermis and is the largest layer of the skin. It contains blood, lymph vessels and nerves.

**Depilatory waxing**   commercially prepared product which is used for the temporary removal of hair root and bulb from the follicle.

**Dermatology**   the study of the skin and its diseases.

**Diabetes mellitus**   a condition which occurs when the pancreas fails to produce sufficient insulin.

**Disinfectant**   a chemical agent which destroys micro-organisms but not usually bacterial spores.

**Double depression**   giving two bursts of current to the follicle during one insertion by depressing the button or foot pedal twice.

**Eczema**   and dermatitis are both terms which may be used to describe the same condition, which varies from a mild to an inflammatory state.

**Electro-epilation**   destruction of hair and follicle by means of an electric current which may be high frequency, galvanic current or a combination of both currents.

**Endocrine gland**   ductless glands situated at specific sites on the body, which secrete hormones directly into the bloodstream, e.g. pituitary gland, thyroid gland.

**Epidermal cord**   slender cord of hair germ cells which enables the retreating follicle to maintain contact with the dermal papilla.

**Epidermis**   protective outer layer of the skin which consists of five layers.

**Epilepsy**   a condition of the nervous system due to disturbance of the brain's electrical activity, which results in convulsive fits.

**Epileptic fit**   temporary disruption to the normal electrical activity of the brain.

**Erythema**   superficial reddening of the skin due to temporary increase of localized blood supply.

**Ethylene oxide**   used as a sterilizing agent.

**Fainting**   temporary loss of consciousness brought about by the reduction of the blood supply to the brain.

**Feeder vein**   refers to the larger vein which supplies smaller capillaries with blood. Term used in association with the treatment of telangiectasia.

**First aid**   immediate assistance given to a casualty in the event of an emergency situation or accident.

**Flash technique**   application of very high intensity of high frequency to the follicle for a fraction of a second.

**Gamma irradiation**   gamma radiation – electro magnetic radiation used for sterilization purposes, for example epilation needles.

**Glutaraldehyde**   chemical preparation used to destroy vegetative bacteria, spores and fungi. The life span of activated glutaraldehyde varies between 14 and 28 days.

**Haemophilia**   an inherited familial condition in which there is excessive bleeding from an injury due to a defect in the blood clotting mechanism.

**Hair**   keratinized structure which grows out of the hair follicle.

**Hair follicle**   sac-like indentation of the epidermis which grows down to the subjacent dermis.

**Hair germ**   consists of undifferentiated cells, which produce new hair when stimulated by circulating hormones and enzyme action.

**Heating pattern**   shape of the heated area of tissue surrounding the needle during the application of high frequency.

**Hepatitis**   inflammation of the liver. An acute infectious, viral disease.

**Herald patch**   refers to the first lesion to appear on the skin at the onset of *Pityriasis Rosea.*

**Herpes Simplex**   acute viral disease characterized by formation of clusters of watery blisters.

**Herpes zoster**   technical name for shingles. It is caused by a virus which is related to the chicken pox virus.

**High frequency**   is produced from an oscillating alternating current of very high frequency and low voltage ranging from 3–30 MHz or 3–30 million cycles per second.

**High frequency field**   the heating pattern radiating from an epilation needle, connected by a wire to a high frequency oscillator. (Shortwave diathermy machine).

**Hirsutism**   masculine pattern of hair growth in women, which is normal in men, caused by increased sensitivity of hair follicles to circulating hormones or by an endocrine disorder.

**HIV**   Human immune deficiency virus which interferes with the immune system, reducing the body's ability to cope effectively with disease or infection.

**Hormone**   complex chemical substance produced by the endocrine glands, which stimulates or inhibits the action of specific glands, organs or tissues.

**Hormone replacement therapy (HRT)**   is the use of natural hormones to replenish the decreased hormone levels which occur during the menopause or after a total hysterectomy.

**Hypertrichosis**   generalized overgrowth of vellus and terminal hairs. Occurs in both sexes. This condition is not hormone dependent but may be due to racial or genetic predisposition.

**Hypothalamus**   part of the mid brain. Situated between the thalamus and the pituitary gland.

**Impetigo**   superficial, contagious, inflammatory disease caused by streptoccocal and staphyloccocal bacteria.

**Infundibulum**   funnel shaped opening to follicle.

**Keloid**   excessive formation of scar tissue at the site of an injury to the skin.

**Keratin**   hard horny substance made up of carbon, hydrogen, sulphur, oxygen and nitrogen; occurs in hair, nails and stratum corneum.

**Keratogenous zone**   area where keratinization takes place in the hair follicle.

**Lye**   is the popular name given to sodium hydroxide.

**Malignant**   severe or threatening to life. The term is applied to any virulent condition which tends to go from bad to worse. Often refers to a cancerous condition.

**Menopause**   the period at which a woman's menstrual cycle stops.

**Menstrual cycle**   usually a 28 day hormonal cycle commencing at puberty, normally ending at the menopause, with a natural interruption during pregnancy.

**Moisture gradient**   refers to the moisture content in the different layers of the skin.

**Oedema**   accumulation of water/fluid in the tissues.

**Ovary**   small endocrine gland which forms part of the female reproductive organs. The ovary produces ova (eggs), oestrogen and progesterone.

**Pain threshold**   the level of stimulation to free nerve endings that can be comfortably tolerated by the individual.

**Pancreas**   large elongated glandular organ with exocrine and endocrine functions. Situated in the curve of the duodenum, behind the stomach.

**Parathyroid glands**   are four small glands embedded in the surfaces of the thyroid gland. Their hormones are responsible for maintaining calcium levels in the blood.

**Pilary canal**   consists of the upper third portion of the outer root sheath, which extends above the entrance of the sebaceous gland.

**Pilo-sebaceous unit**   formed from the hair follicle and the sebaceous gland.

**Pituitary gland**   known as the master gland of the endocrine system due to its influence on the other endocrine glands. Produces trophic hormones.

**Pityriasis rosea**   self limiting skin disease with no known cause. Normally runs its course within six weeks.

**Plucking**   mechanical removal of an individual hair by means of a pair of tweezers. Also known as tweezing.

**Premenstrual tension (PMT)**   is the name given to a collection of mental and physical symptoms, due to hormonal changes, which occur for up to ten days before menstruation.

**Professional ethics**   code of conduct or standards of behaviour practised by the professional electrolysist in relation to clients, colleagues, the medical profession and professional associations.

**Psoriasis**   chronic, inflammatory, non-contagious condition of the skin.

**Puberty**   the period of change from childhood to adolescence when the sex glands become active.

**Public relations (PR)**   is concerned with promoting a business through image, presentation and personal contact.

**Recovery position**   is used to keep a casualty's air passages open and free from obstruction, particularly when the casualty is unconscious.

**Rhinophyma**   a condition of the nose which shows thickening of the skin and enlargement of skin tissues. Usually a high colour is present.

**Rosacea**   a chronic skin disease of the face; characterized by redness and the formation of pustules. Coarsening of the skin also occurs.

**Sebaceous cyst**   round, nodular lesion with a smooth shiny surface which develops from a sebaceous gland.

**Sebaceous glands**   are attached to hair follicles. Their function is to produce sebum.

**Sepsis**   presence of infection due to germs or micro-organisms.

**Shock**   disturbance of the emotions, or state of bodily collapse due to severe bleeding, burns, fright, unpleasant news or electrical shock.

**Sodium hydroxide**   caustic chemical substance, produced during galvanic electrolysis. Destroys tissue by chemical action. Also known as lye.

**Spider naevus**   collection of telangiectasia which radiate from a central papule.

**Sterilization**   process used to achieve total destruction of all living organisms and spores.

**Sudoriferous gland**   more commonly referred to as sweat gland. Found all over the body. The function of these glands is to produce sweat which regulates body heat and eliminates waste products.

**Sugaring**   commercial substance based on lemon juice, sugar and water which removes hair in a similar manner to waxing when applied to the skin.

**Telangiectasis**   dilation of small blood vessels in the skin. Often referred to as broken veins, red veins, thread veins, or dilated capillaries.

**Telogen**   final stage of hair growth cycle, which follows on from catagen.

**Thyroid gland**   largest endocrine gland situated in the neck. Its secretion controls metabolism and body growth.

**Transsexual**   a person who feels strongly that he/she is trapped in the wrong biological body.

**Units of lye**   tenths of a milliamp × times in seconds = units of lye. i.e. one tenth of a milliamp of dc flowing for one second produces one unit of lye.

**Urticaria**   development of red wheals which may later become white. Lesions appear rapidly and disappear within minutes over a number of hours.

**VAT**   refers to value added tax, which is levied on most business transactions which take place within the Economic European Community (EEC), UK and Isle of Man.

**Vitiligo**   name used to describe lack of pigmentation in the skin.

**Warts**   viral infection. Well defined, benign tumours which vary in size.

# Bibliography

*Structure and Function of the Skin*, W. Montagna and Ellis.

*Essential Notions of Black Skin*, H. Pierantoni.

*Human Hairgrowth in Health and Disease*, David Ferriman.

*Hair Research 1981, Status and Future Aspects*, edited by C.E. Orfanos, W. Montagna and G. Stuttgen.

*Advances in Biology of Skin and Hair Growth*, Montagna and Dobson, Pergamon Press.

*Gray's Anatomy*, The Classic Collector's edition.

*The Principles and Practise of Hairdressing*, Leo Palladino.

*The Cause and Management of Hirsutism*, edited by R.B. Greenblatt, V.B. Mahesh and R.D. Gambrell.

*International Hair Route Magazine*.

*Basic Knowledge of Esthetiques*, Humbert Pierantoni.

*Anatomy and Physiology*, Evelyn Pearce.

*The Hirsute Female*, R.B. Greenblatt.

*Endocrinology*, Small-Clarke-Williams, Heinemann.

*Hormones and the Body*, A Stuart Mason, Pelican.

*Electrolysis, Thermolysis and the Blend*, Hinkle and Lind.

*Lecture Notes on Dermatology 1990*, Graham-Brown and Burns, Blackwell.

*No Change*, Wendy Cooper, 1990.

*Dermatology*, Lionel Fry, Updated edition.

*Dermatology*, P Hall-Smith, R.I. Cairns and R.L.B. Beare, 2nd edition, CLS.

*The Beauty Salon and its Equipment*, John Simmons, MacMillan, 1989.

*Clayton's Electrotherapy*, 8th edition, Forster and Palastanga, Bailliere Tindall.

*Ross & Wilson Anatomy and Physiology*, 7th edition, Kathleen, J.W. Wilson, Churchill Livingstone.

*Principles of Electrology and Shortwave Epilation*, edited by Arthur Mahler, 1986.

*Electrolysis Exam Review*, John Fantz.

*The Fantz Guide to Electrolysis*, John Fantz, Laurel Publication, 1983.

*Health and Beauty Therapy – A Practical Approach for NVQ Level 3*, Dawn Mernagh and Jennifer Cartwright, Stanley Thornes (Publishers) Ltd, 1995.

*CIBTAC NVQ/SVQ Guide Level 3*, Electrical Epilation, 1994.

*Managing the Menopause II – a guide to HRT*, Cathy Read, Edited by David Sturdee.

*The Blend*, Michael Bono, 1995.

*Body Shock, The Truth about Changing Sex*, Liz Hodgkinson.

*Guidelines for Transsexuals Male to Female and Female to Male*, SHAFT.

*Speech Pathology Considerations in the Management of Transsexualism*, Jennifer Oates and Georgia Dacakis.

*Science for the Beauty Therapist*, John Rounce, Stanley Thornes.

*Roxburgh's Common Skin Diseases*, 15th edition, John D. Kirby, H.K. Lewis & Co, London, 1986.

*Acne Update Postgraduate Series*, W.J. Cunliffe.

*Eczema & Psoriasis Update Postgraduate Series*, R.H. Champion.

*The Biology of Hair Growth*, W. Montagna and Ellis.

*First-Aid Manual,* St John Ambulance The British Red Cross Society, St Andrews Association, 5th edition, 1987.

*Hygienic Skin Piercing*, Dr Noah, 1988.

*Parr's Concise Medical Encyclopaedia*, John Anthony Parr and Robert A. Young, Elsevier, 1971.

*The VAT Guide,* (revised 1987), HM Customs and Excise.

*Inland Revenue Publications November 1988*, Leaflets IR57, IR109.

*Current Law Statutes*, annotated 1963.

*Current Law Statutes*, annotated 1974.

*Current Law Statutes*, annotated 1982.

*Croner's Health and Safety at Work*, 1990.

*National Westminster Bank PLC, Guide for small businesses.*

*Department of Heath and Social Security Leaflets FB30, NI40, NI41.*

*Sterilisation and Hygiene*, W.G. Peberdy, Stanley Thornes, 1988.

Inland Revenue Publications – *Tax, Guide to self-assessment for the self-employed.*

Data Protection Act 1984, *The Guidelines 3rd Series*, November 1994, Office of the Data Protection registrar.

## Professional publication

International Hair Route Magazine
Suite 212
106 Lakeshore Road East
Mississauga
Ontario L5G 1ES
Canada
Tel: 001-905-271-0339; fax: 001-905-271-9748

# Professional associations

British Association of Electrolysists Ltd
8 Chaul End Road
Caddington
Beds LV1 4AS
Tel: 01582-487743

Institute of Electrolysis
138 Downs Barn Boulevard
Downs Barn
Milton Keynes MK14 7RP
Tel/fax: 01908–695–297

Membership of the above associations may be gained by demonstrating practical skills to a board of examiners and successfully sitting a theory paper.

British Association of Beauty Therapy and Cosmetology
Parabola House
Parabola Road
Cheltenham
Glos G150 3AH
Tel: 01242-570284; fax: 01242-222177

American Electrology Association
106 Oak Ridge Road
Trumbull CT0 6611

Canadian Organization of Professional Electrologists
170 St George Street
Suite 408
Toronto
Ontario M5R 2M8
Canada

Federation of Canadian Electrolysis Associations
PO Box 1513
Station B, Mississauga
Ontario L4Y 4G2
Canada

International Guild of Professional Electrologists Inc
Professional Building, Suite C
202 Boulevard
High Point
North Carolina
USA 27260

Society of Clinical and Medical Electrologists Inc
PO Box 52
Killeen
Texas
USA 76540

# Examination boards in the UK

British Association of Electrolysists Ltd
8 Chaul End Road
Caddington
Beds LU1 4AS
Tel: 01582-487743

Institute of Electrolysis
138 Downs Barn Boulevard
Downs Barn
Milton Keynes MK14 7RP

The above boards are concerned specifically with electrical epilation. The following boards examine subjects relating to beauty therapy in conjunction with electrical epilation.

Confederation of International Beauty Therapy and Cosmetology
Parabole House
Parabola Road
Cheltenham
Glos GL50 3AH
Tel: 01242-570284

City and Guilds of London Institute
46 Britannia Street
London WC1X 9RG

International Health and Beauty Council
PO Box 36
Arundel
West Sussex BN18 0SW

Business and Technical Education Council
(BTEC)
Tavistock House South
Entrance D
Tavistock Square
London
WC1H 9LG

# Index

—